Machine Learning and Optimization Frameworks for Women's Nutritional Health

Somya

Table of Contents

List of Tables

List of Figures

LIST OF ABBREVIATIONS

AI	-	Artificial Intelligence
ANN	-	Artificial Neural Network
BiGRU	-	Bidirectional Gated Recurrent Unit
CNN	-	Convolutional Neural Network
CF	-	Collaborative Filtering
DL	-	Deep Learning
DNN	-	Deep Neural Network
DT	-	Decision Tree
EDA	-	Exploratory Data Analysis
F1-Score	-	Harmonic Mean of Precision and Recall
FCM	-	Fuzzy C-Means
FSH	-	Follicle-Stimulating Hormone
GGOA	-	Greylag Goose Optimization Algorithm
HABi-ConGRNet	-	Hybrid Attention-Based Bidirectional GRU Network
HPO Axis	-	Hypothalamic–Pituitary–Ovarian Axis
HRT	-	Hormone Replacement Therapy
IOT	-	Internet of Things
KNN	-	K-Nearest Neighbors
LH	-	Luteinizing Hormone
LSAENet	-	Layered Sparse Autoencoder Network
LSTM	-	Long Short-Term Memory
ML	-	Machine Learning
OL	-	Opposition Learning
OL-RPO	-	Opposition Learning-Based Red Panda Optimization
PCA	-	Principal Component Analysis
PMS	-	Premenstrual Syndrome
PMDD	-	Premenstrual Dysphoric Disorder

RBF	-	Radial Basis Function
RF	-	Random Forest
RNN	-	Recurrent Neural Network
ROC	-	Receiver Operating Characteristic
RPO	-	Red Panda Optimization
SVM	-	Support Vector Machine
TP	-	True Positive
TN	-	True Negative
FP	-	False Positive
FN	-	False Negative
ViT	-	Vision Transformer
XGBoost	-	Extreme Gradient Boosting
WHO	-	World Health Organization

CHAPTER 1

INTRODUCTION

1.1 AN OVERVIEW OF WOMEN'S REPRODUCTIVE LIFECYCLE AND NUTRITIONAL NEEDS

Biological and hormonal fluctuations in the reproductive lifecycle have a strong impact on women health and are divided into three major stages: menarche (commencing of menstruation), menstrual cycle, and menopause. Every stage has its own nutritional requirements and health care issues and special dietary methods are needed. Although the traditional rules provide some general guidelines, they may not represent the personal differences in physiology, lifestyle, genetics, and environment. Recent achievements in Artificial Intelligence (AI), machine learning, and optimization methods allow building individual nutrition systems that adjust to the changing needs of the women dynamically. This part gives a summary of the reproductive lifecycle and AI-based frameworks that were created in this thesis to respond to such challenges in figure 1.1.

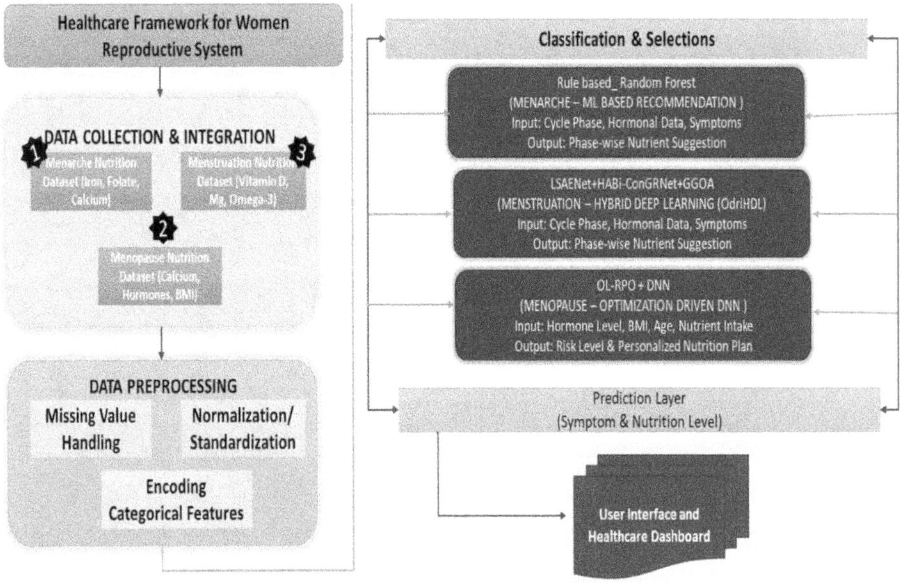

Figure 1.1. Healthcare Framework

1.1.1 PERSONALIZED NUTRITION FOR ADOLESCENT GIRLS AT MENARCHE USING MACHINE LEARNING

The menarche is the beginning of reproductive maturity which normally starts between 10 to 15. At this phase, hormonal shifts cause some symptoms like abdominal cramps, irregular cycles, fatigue and mood swings. There is widespread deficiency of nutrients particularly iron, folate, calcium, and protein, and it has been reported in the world that more than half of the teenage girls are anaemic. The module of the research uses the machine learning models (Rule based Random Forest, K-Nearest Neighbors, XGBoost) in determining the severity of symptoms and prescribing dietary changes. Using clinical and nutritional datasets, the system was able to identify 92% of the cases and this illustrates the promise of AI in the treatment of dietary intervention at the initial stages of the condition in figure1.2. This will make sure that the adolescent girls are provided with individualized nutrition strategies that will lead to better health outcomes and reproductive wellness in the long term.

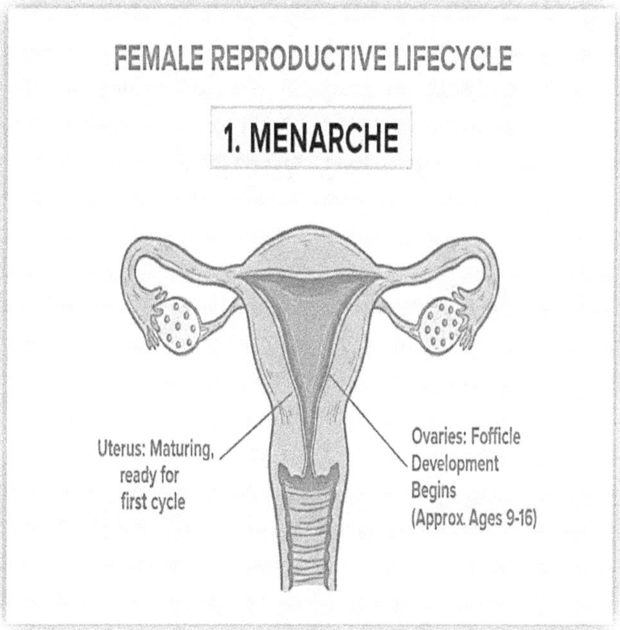

Figure 1.2. Female Reproductive System Menarche

1.1.2 HYBRID GREYLAG GOOSE WITH LAYERED SPARSE NETWORK FOR WOMEN'S NUTRITION DURING MENSTRUAL CYCLE

The menstrual cycle is broken down into four stages, namely, follicular, ovulation, luteal, and menstrual in figure 1.3. A different set of nutritional needs is needed at every stage, e.g. iron and vitamin B6 are essential at the point of menstruation, and calcium, magnesium and omega-3 fatty acids can help relieve the symptoms of PMS in the luteal phase. According to the studies, almost 70 percent of women have unmanaged PMS symptoms, which result in a lower quality of life. In this module, a hybrid AI architecture is presented that incorporates both Layered Sparse Autoencoder (LSAENet) and Hybrid Attention-based BiGRU Network (HABi-ConGRNet) that is optimized with Greylag Goose Optimization Algorithm (GGOA). The model is dynamic to changes that occur at different phases and has a 97.5% accuracy in nutrition suggestions. The model shows that AI-driven models can be used to manage complex, cyclical nutritional requirements.

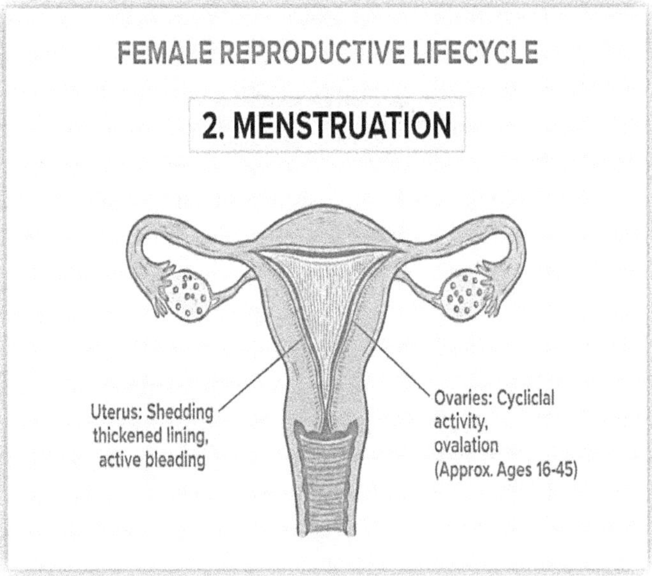

Figure 1.3. Female Reproductive System Menstruation

1.1.3 OPPOSITION LEARNING-BASED RED PANDA OPTIMIZATION FOR MENOPAUSAL NUTRITION INTELLIGENCE

Menopause is a condition that usually starts at the age of 45-55 and is characterized by the decreasing levels of estrogen that predisposes a person to osteoporosis, heart diseases, obesity, and mood swings in figure 1.4. It has been found out that 1 out of every 3 postmenopausal women has osteoporosis, also cardiovascular complications are much higher than that of premenopausal women. In order to overcome these issues, this module presents an Opposition Learning-Red Panda Optimization (OL-RPO) algorithm together with a Deep Neural Network (DNN). The framework has 98.1% accuracy by using advanced feature selection of high-dimensional nutritional and clinical data and 45.7 reduction of irrelevant feature. The system gives specific nutrition advice on calcium, vitamin D, protein, and omega-3 fatty acids which maximizes the health results in the long-term.

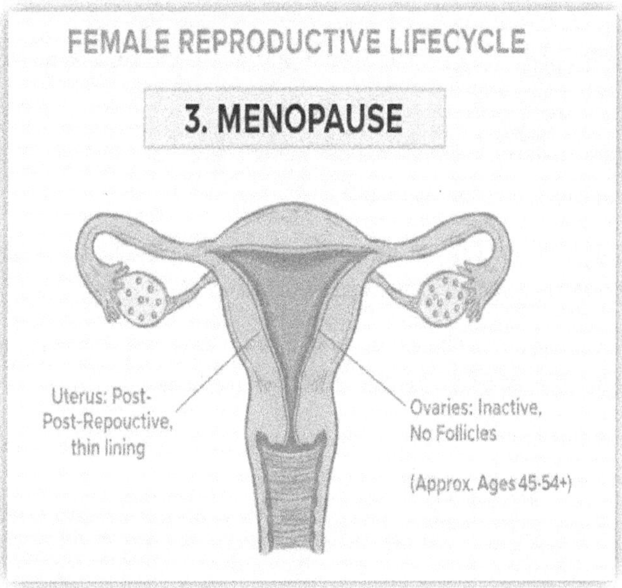

Figure 1.4. Female Reproductive System Menopause

1.2 THE ROLE OF ARTIFICIAL INTELLIGENCE IN PRECISION NUTRITION FOR WOMEN'S HEALTHCARE

AI has a revolutionary promise in the healthcare sector since it can examine vast, intricate databases comprising dietary habits, clinical data, and lifestyle information. In contrast to the conventional means, AI has the ability to reveal latent patterns and nonlinear connections between nutrition and health. Machine learning models predict trends of symptoms whereas deep learning models predict intricate temporal interdependence across reproductive phases. Bio-inspired optimization also improves on accuracy with feature selection and parameter optimization. Combining these approaches, AI-assisted precision nutrition will go beyond the one-size-fits-all recommendation, providing accessible evidence-based interventions based on each phase of the reproductive lifecycle of a woman. This renders AI an effective instrument in the process of closing the divide between clinical healthcare and customized dietary control.

1.2.1 CHALLENGES IN WOMEN'S NUTRITION AND THE NEED FOR AN AI-BASED FRAMEWORK

Although there have been improvements toward women healthcare, a number of challenges still exist:

- Generalized Guidelines: Traditional diet schemes do not consider the idea of biological diversity, which causes their differing results.
- High rate of Nutritional Deficits: Iron-deficiency anemia, calcium deficiency and vitamin D deficiency are common in women in many parts of the world.
- Multidimensional Data: Nutritional and clinical data are complex, and it would be challenging to analyze them using standard statistical methods.
- Absence of Customisation: The existing systems can very seldom be phase- or stage-specific to the differences in reproductive health of women.

CHAPTER 2

AIM AND OBJECTIVE

2.1 PROBLEM IDENTIFICATION

Every stage of the reproductive life cycle of a woman, the menarche, menstrual phases, and menopause, come with their own nutrition and health problems. During menarche, adolescent girls often experience irregular periods, iron deficiency, anemia and fatigue. The conditions that an individual experiences during the menstrual cycle due to the varying hormone levels include cramps, mood swings and premenstrual syndrome (PMS). Low estrogen levels in menopause increase the risks of osteoporosis, cardiovascular disease, obesity and metabolic disorders. Traditional nutrition policies tend to be universal and fixed, and they give general recommendations like taking more calcium or iron. Nonetheless, they do not meet the changing and stage-specific needs of women that result in uneven healthcare outcomes. Moreover, the nutritional and clinical data are complex and have a large number of variables (macronutrients, micronutrients, biomarkers, lifestyle factors, etc.) that cannot be easily processed using conventional approaches. This study determines the missing fundamental link between the personalized, adaptive, and clinically interpretable nutrition systems. In the absence of the use of sophisticated AI and optimization algorithms, women cannot be served by the existing models of healthcare that fail to consider the nutritional needs at each stage. This proposed work will address these issues by creating an integrated AI-driven platform that will be able to provide accuracy in the nutrition recommendation throughout the reproductive lifecycle.

2.2 MOTIVATION

Healthcare amongst women is an international agenda and nutrition has been posed as a pillar of lifetime health. The World Health Organization (WHO) reports that over 500 million women have iron-deficiency anemia and that adolescents have a high prevalence. More than 70 percent of women have PMS-related symptoms, which are likely to be inadequately addressed with the help of generic interventions. A third of postmenopausal women are affected with osteoporosis, and millions of women are facing cardiovascular and metabolic complications all over the world.

Although such statistics are alarming, the nutrition strategies are generic and do not take into consideration individual differences in physiology, lifestyle and genetic predisposition. The emergence of Artificial Intelligence (AI), machine learning, deep learning, and bio-inspired optimization offers us a chance to make this gap by offering stage-specific, individualized and adaptive nutrition solutions.

This study is driven by the fact that there is a need to:

- Improve the life of women throughout their reproductive years.
- Offer AI-powered medical systems capable of meeting the changing nutritional needs.
- Minimized risks in the long-term, based on nutritional deficiencies and disorders related to lifestyle.
- Work towards global health equity by working on the United Nations Sustainable Development Goal 3: Good Health and Well-Being.

2.3 AIM AND OBJECTIVE

Construct and implement an Artificial Intelligence-Based Precision Nutrition and Healthcare Framework that provides individualised, stage-specific, and clinically interpretable guidance for women across the reproductive lifespan.

Objectives:

- To develop machine learning models for forecasting symptoms and offering nutritional guidance for adolescent girls experiencing menarche.
- To provide a hybrid deep learning and optimization framework for phase-specific nutritional recommendations throughout the menstrual cycle.
- To propose an Opposition Learning-Red Panda Optimization (OL-RPO) augmented deep learning model for precision nutrition in menopause.
- To consolidate all three models obsessed by a cohesive AI-driven healthcare outline including the female reproductive period.
- To assess system performance utilising benchmark datasets and measures such as accuracy, precision, recall, F1-score, feature reduction, and accomplishment duration.

2.4 SIGNIFICANCE OF THE STUDY

This research advances women's healthcare, computational intelligence, and personalized medicine in several respects:

- Healthcare Impact: Offers tailored nutritional recommendations for symptom management and the avoidance of chronic problems such as anaemia, premenstrual syndrome, osteoporosis, and cardiovascular disease.
- Technological Innovation: Introduces innovative AI frameworks that integrate machine learning, deep learning, and bio-inspired optimisation, hence improving accuracy and feature selection.
- Academic Contribution: Develops benchmark models exhibiting excellent accuracy (92%–98.1%) throughout reproductive phases, enhancing the literature on AI-driven healthcare.
- Societal Significance: Equips women with practical nutritional knowledge, enhancing health outcomes and bolstering global efforts for women's well-being.

2.5 SCOPE OF THE STUDY

The scope of this thesis is limited to the application of AI techniques for precision nutrition and healthcare across the reproductive lifecycle. It focuses on three key stages: menarche, menstrual cycle, and menopause.

- Inclusions:
    - Development of stage-specific models using ML, DL, and optimization.
    - Evaluation using benchmark datasets and standard performance metrics.
    - Integration into a unified AI-driven precision nutrition framework.
- Exclusions / Limitations:
    - Real-time clinical trials and patient-specific data collection are beyond scope.
    - IoT-based wearable integrations are proposed as future work but not implemented.
    - Cultural and geographical variations in dietary patterns may not be fully represented.

2.6 THESIS ORGANIZATION

- Chapter 1 – Introduction Gives a summary of the research problem, motivation, aim and objectives, significance, scope and general thesis structure. It notes the necessity of an AI-powered accuracy nutrition/healthcare platform in women throughout their reproductive lifecycle.
- Chapter 2 – Literature Review Survey literature on the topic of nutrition, reproductive health, and AI-based care platforms in women. It mentions the flaws of traditional nutritional methods, explains how machine learning, deep learning, and optimization can be applied to healthcare, and specifies the research opportunities discussed in this paper.
- Chapter 3: An Intelligent Machine Learning-Based Personalized Nutrition Recommendation of Adolescent Menarche Girls. Introduces the first component of the framework, and uses machine learning models, including Rule based Random Forest, K-Nearest Neighbors (KNN), and XGBoost, to predict symptom severity and make custom nutritional advice to adolescent girls going through menarche.
- Chapter 4- Hybrid Greylag Goose with Layered Sparse Network of Women Nutrition Suggestions during Menstrual Cycle. A description of the second module, which presents a Hybrid Deep Learning model that is a combination of Layered Sparse Autoencoder (LSAENet), Hybrid Attention-based BiGRU (HABi-ConGRNet), and Greylag Goose Optimization Algorithm (GGOA). The module provides the nutrition advice at the individual phases of the menstrual cycle.
- Chapter 5- Optimalization techniques of the nutritional recommendation during menopause using red panda optimization. Describes the third module, using an Opposition Learning based Red Panda Optimization (OL-RPO) algorithm with a Deep Neural Network (DNN). This method improves the choice of features in high dimensional data and gives accurate nutrition advice to the menopausal women.
- Chapter 6- Gives experimental findings, performance review, and comparison of all the three modules. It also shows that the proposed models are effective in terms of accuracy, precision, recall, F1-score, feature reduction, and execution time, as well as confirms the clinical importance of the entire framework.
- Chapter 7- Conclusions and Future Work. Provides a summary of the principal contributions of the study, which encompass the development of a unified AI-driven system for precision nutrition and healthcare in women. It also delineates restrictions and prospective

avenues for incorporating real-time interaction with the Internet of Things, wearable devices, and cloud-based healthcare systems.

2.7 SUMMARY

This chapter developed a background of the study including the necessity of an artificial intelligent operated precision nutrition and healthcare model among women throughout the reproductive lifecycle. It highlighted the special nutritional issues of women at menarche, menstrual cycle and during menopause and the drawbacks of traditional and generalized diets. The chapter has given the problem identification supported with the world healthcare statistics, and determination of the motivation of creating the artificial intelligent based personalized based, and clinically interpretable nutrition solutions. The goal and the purpose were clearly stipulated with three autonomous but interdependent modules of different reproductive phases. The importance of the research was presented in connection to healthcare, technological innovation, contribution to the academic field, and the impact on society. The research boundaries, applications, and future extensions of the framework were understood through the scope of the research. Lastly, the organization of the thesis offered an overview of the work, giving a layout of how the ideas moved in the literature review up to how models were developed, experimentally validated, results and conclusions.

CHAPTER 3

LITERATURE REVIEW

3.1 INTRODUCTION

Provides an in-depth assessment of the biological, psychosocial, and technological determinants of female reproductive health throughout the life course. The beginning of puberty is a very crucial phase in the process of female development, which is marked by the hormones changes that govern the development of the secondary sexual organs, development of the reproductive organs and the initiation of the menstrual cycles. The genetic and physiological factors affecting these processes are not only influenced by the environment but also predisposed by early life experiences, nutrition and psychosocial environment. The nutritional status such as the intake of macro and micronutrients is central in regulating the time of menarche, the regularity of menstruation and reproductive functioning. Moreover, menstrual health is influenced by diseases like anemia, abnormal cycles, hormonal disorders, and such diseases as polycystic ovary syndrome (PCOS). In addition to the biological processes, psychosocial and cultural processes, such as education, awareness, and hygiene practices, have a critical influence on the health of menstruation and the possibility of adolescent girls to control menstruation safely and confidently.

The literature also highlights the importance of lifestyle, dietary habits and nutrient intake in promoting reproductive and menstrual health. Menstrual irregularities, menstrual pain, and related metabolic effects have been attributed to variations in energy intake, deficiency of some micronutrients, and eating habits. These health outcomes can be further exacerbated by the psychosocial aspects of menstruation such as stress, fear and the stigma process and hence holistic methods that integrates education, behavioral and nutritional support are important. During adulthood reproductive health still reacts in response to diet, physical activity and lifestyle behavior with cumulative effects apparent in fertility, reproductive longevity, and menopausal transitions. Menopause as the natural replacement of reproductive ability is accompanied by physiological, psychological, and metabolic alterations, which need attentive monitoring and control. Nutritional therapy, lifestyle change and specific health care are essential in the relief of menopausal symptoms, cardiovascular and bone health and in the enhancement of living quality.

Recent advancements in computational technologies revolutionized women's reproductive health research. AI-driven models, encompassing predictive algorithms, wearable health monitoring devices, and deep learning architectures and ensemble models, have been utilised to monitor menstrual cycles, anticipate symptom patterns, and deliver personalized dietary and lifestyle recommendations. These technologies provide continuous, real-time monitoring of physiological indicators, providing women with meaningful insights into their reproductive health and enhancing clinical decision-making. AI-driven recommender systems, health chatbots, and femtech applications offer personalized advice on diet, hormonal fluctuations, and symptom management, effectively connecting conventional healthcare delivery with technology-facilitated self-care. Integrating computer models with nutritional and lifestyle data facilitates precision health strategies, ensuring therapies are customised to each individual's distinct reproductive profile and life stage.

3.2 BIOLOGICAL BASIS OF PUBERTY, MENSTRUAL CYCLE, AND REPRODUCTIVE AGING

The female reproductive health is the lifelong biological continuum in which pubertal maturation leads to cyclic reproductive functioning, and reproductive senescence is the end of biological process. The hypothalamic-pituitary-ovarian (HPO) axis controls these stages and incorporates neuroendocrine cues with metabolic, environmental, and psychosocial stimuli. It is important to understand this continuum since the imbalances at each level can result in ripple effects on the physical, psychological and metabolic health in the long run.

Puberty is a significant neuroendocrine restructuring, which is marked by the reinstitution of gonadotropin-releasing hormone (GnRH) pulsatility. This triggering causes downstream release of luteinizing hormone (LH) and follicle-stimulating hormone (FSH) to result in ovarian steroidogenesis and secondary sexual characteristics formation. As pointed out by Howard (2021), the interpretation of pubertal hormones is complicated because the factors are overlapping, developmental, circadian, or environmental. Late puberty hormonal changes tend to complicate clinical diagnosis especially when it comes to differentiating between a normal change in development and a pathological endocrine disturbance. Present-day testimony points out the fact that the timing of puberty is not entirely genetically encoded. Hamlat et al. (2023) established that childhood adversity in the form of socioeconomic instability, stress in the household, and food insecurity boosts pubertal onset. Their results are in favor of life-history theory which says that biological systems respond to perceived environmental threats by adapting reproductive timing. This acceleration can heighten the susceptibility of mental illness, metabolic illness and premature reproductive exposure. Preparedness to education is of key buffering significance to this transition. The results indicated by Mohammed Abd El Aliem et al. (2023) demonstrated that structured instructional guidelines are associated with a high level of improvement in the knowledge related to puberty, anxiety decrease, and adaptive behavior in adolescents. Their results highlight the significance of a biological education and psychosocial support programs in the period of transitioning to puberty.

One of the major modulators of pubertal development is nutrition. Hypothalamic GnRH-signaling is sensitive to adequate energy supply, micronutrient adequacy, and fat composition in the body. Recent studies by Christanti and Syafiq (2023) found that the relationship between diets rich in fiber, phytoestrogens, and micronutrients and age at menarche was positive, as diets rich in these components can delay menarche by effecting adiposity and estrogen metabolism. On the other hand, reproductive maturation may be slowed down by nutritional deprivation or chronic illness. Di Maio et al. (2023) also explored the subject of transfusion-dependent thalassemia and found that these individuals experience delayed menarche, menstrual abnormalities, and diminished ovarian reserve. The effects of chronic anemia and iron overload and endocrine dysfunction ultimately affect development of the normal ovary, which demonstrates how sensitive the reproductive axis is to systemic disease. Also, the contribution of cognition and evolutionary biology to reproductive timing has been noted. Yong and Kanazawa (2025) suggested relationships among intelligence, the age of puberty and reproductive strategies, and that the later maturation can be correlated with longer educational investment and changes in fertility behavior. Though highly contentious, these views put across the point that puberty is influenced by both biological ability and environmental adaptation.

Menarche is followed by the appearance of menstrual cycle, which is a regular endocrine process indicating the coordination of ovaries and uterus. A detailed clinical approach was presented by Itriyeva (2022) who outlined follicular and ovulatory phases as well as luteal phases that have a characteristic hormonal makeup. During the follicular and luteal phases, estradiol and progesterone respectively would help in the proliferation of the endometria and ready the uterus to be implanted. Correct determination of menstrual phases is imperative in the study and practice. Gloe et al. (2023) have cited methodological weaknesses in the determination of the cycle phases such as use of self-reporting and calendar estimates. All these modifications were pushed by them to adopt the multimodal designs that constituted of hormonal tests, basal body temperature, and digital trackers to achieve accuracy.

Regularity of the menstrual cycle is now being viewed as a sign of overall wellness. According to Vladimirovna et al. (2023) and Rakhimova (2023), stress, nutritional imbalance, an endocrine imbalance, and lifestyle are among the primary causes of menstrual cycle disruptions. Such upsets usually represent a metabolic or personal psychological dysfunction and not a discrete gynaecologic pathology. Teenage is a highly vulnerable stage. As stated by Klusmann et al. (2023), menstrual cycles in adolescents can never be predictable because the HPO axis is still maturing. Medicalizing normal variation can cause unwarranted treatment, and under medicalizing chronic abnormality can result in a delay in the diagnosis of endocrine diseases like polycystic ovary syndrome (PCOS). Menstrual patterns are predictive of the risk of chronic disease across the lifespan. Cunningham et al. (2024) reported longitudinal variations in the length of the cycle, variability, and burden of symptoms since adolescence to perimenopause. Wang et al. (2022) showed that long-term menstrual irregularity is linked to a high risk of cardiovascular disease, which supports the idea that menstrual health is a portal into systemic physiology. Vollmar et al. (2025) went a step ahead and suggested the menstrual cycle to be a vital sign, just as is the case with heart rate or blood pressure. Such framing would help the clinicians and researchers consider menstrual data as part of a normal health examination and not reproductive niche.

The features of reproductive aging include the reduction in follicular reserve, changed steroidogenesis, and the subsequent termination of menstruation. Xing et al. (2023) showed that premature menopause is related to high mortality rates which are all cause mortality, and the focus of the study is on the long-term effects of early ovarian failure. Wang et al. (2023) have associated the short period of reproduction with the increase in the symptoms of depression, which underscores the mental consequences of reproductive aging. Genomic instability, mitochondrial dysfunction and inflammatory signaling are the molecular mechanisms involved in ovarian aging. Benayoun et al. (2025) investigated these processes and found epigenetic markers that are related to ovarian senescence. Xu et al. (2025) proposed OvaRePred ovarian aging clock, which is an AI-based framework that can precisely predict reproductive aging pathways using hormonal and molecular measurements. There is a heightened psycho neuroendocrine vulnerability in perimenopause. According to Schweizer-Schubert et al. (2025), this transition is characterized by dysregulation of the stress hormones, as well as neurotransmitter systems. In their other study, Zuo et al. (2025) also investigated postmenopausal depression and found that reproductive history was a strong predictor of mental health in adulthood.

3.3 MENSTRUAL HEALTH, HYGIENE, NUTRITION AND PSYCHOSOCIAL FACTORS ACROSS THE FEMALE LIFE COURSE

The World Health Organization defines menstrual health as a total physical, mental and social wellness with respect to the menstrual cycle. The viewpoint goes beyond a narrow biomedical understanding as it incorporates the dignity, comfort, safety and autonomy. This paradigm was reinforced by Vollmar et al. (2025) who offered menstrual patterns as the valuable sign as they say that this cycle regularity, bleeding features, and symptom burden can give an insight about the cardiometabolic and endocrine and mental health. The factors that influence menstrual health are age, nutritional status, socioeconomic conditions, cultural beliefs and availability of sanitation facilities. Teenagers are especially vulnerable because of their lack of knowledge, stigma, and lack of support Mohammed Abd El Aliem et al. (2023). Stress in work life, dietary changes and reproductive experiences in adulthood also moderate menstrual experiences Cunningham et al. (2024).

Management of menstrual hygiene has been defined as the use of clean materials to absorb menstrual blood, the capacity to replace these materials in privacy where they need it frequently, the ability to use soap and water in washing and safe disposal of used products. Regardless of the basic necessity, MHM is a major health issue in countries with low and middle income. Liberty et al. (2023) explored the innovations in menstrual technology and pointed to the inequality in the access to safe, affordable, and sustainable products. Although new inventions like menstrual cups and reusable pads have long term advantages, their use is limited by cultural resistance, education and infrastructural factors. Research in South Asia and Sub-Saharan Africa document that girls usually do not go to school during their menstrual period because of lack of sanitation facilities as well as because of fear of embarrassment.

Nutrition has been at the center of the regulation of menstrual cycles, the severity of symptoms and overall reproductive health. Macronutrients have been shown to maintain balance of energy if consumed adequately, whereas micronutrients like iron, calcium, magnesium, zinc, and B6 and D are required to synthesize hormones and support neuromuscular activity. Nagata et al. (2023) have shown that there is a powerful correlation between the food insecurity and the binge eating disorder at the time of early adolescence, and binge eating disorder has effects cascading through to the menstrual irregularity. Nutritional instability interferes with leptin signaling, disturbs gonadotropin secretion, and raises cortisol levels and all these factors impair ovulatory events. Among the most common nutritional disorders is iron deficiency anemia that is observed in menstruating individuals. Menstrual bleeding is a heavy one that enhances the loss of iron, which leads to a cyclic effect between menstruation and anemia. As Liberty et al. (2023) stated, menstrual technology innovations cannot be effective only unless they are combined with nutritional interventions and health education. Vegetarian eating habits are becoming popular with regard to the effects on menstrual health. Diets consisting of fruits, vegetables, and whole grains, as reported by Christanti and Syafiq (2023) can help minimize the severity of dysmenorrhea via anti-inflammatory mechanisms.

Menstrual diseases, such as dysmenorrhea, menorrhagia, oligomenorrhea and premenstrual syndrome (PMS) have a severe effect on day-to-day functioning. Dysmenorrhea is one of the major causes of absenteeism in schools and workplaces in the world. Severe menstrual pain is usually accompanied by psychological distress, sleep disturbances and decreased physical activity. According to Vladimirovna et al. (2023), stress and lifestyle imbalance were among the most frequent predictors of menstrual irregularities. Chronic stress triggers hypothalamic-pituitary adrenal axis and inhibits the release of gonadotropin and changes the period of the cycle. Rakhimova (2023) also reported that the current sedentary lifestyle, sleep disorders, and uncontrolled intake of caffeine worsen symptoms of menstruation. Premenstrual dysphoric disorder (PMDD) is a serious type of PMS, which is accompanied by mood swings, irritability, and depressed mood. Schweizer-Schubert et al. (2025) emphasized the neuroendocrine sensitivity to hormonal variations as one of the major processes that contribute to PMDD and connects the variation in reproductive hormones with serotonergic imbalances.

Menstruation is very interwoven with sociocultural constructs that conceptualize attitudes, behavior, and self-esteem. In most societies, menstruation is a culture of shamefulness, impurity and secretive nature. Such stigmatization has adverse mental health and health-seeking behavior. Mohammed Abd El Aliem et al. (2023) proved that, with the use of educational intervention methods, menstrual-related anxiety and misperceptions in teenagers can be decreased significantly. The knowledge empowerment will help in the development of a positive body image, better hygiene practices, and prompt medical consultation. There are also gender norms that affect the menstrual experiences in adulthood. Poor working conditions including absence of menstrual accommodations facilitate presenteeism and low productivity. Cunningham et al. argued in favor of menstrual-inclusive health policies according to which menstruation is a physiological process and not a secret and inconvenient inconvenience (2024).

The emergence of digital menstrual tracking apps has changed self-management during menstruation. These applications allow users to track cycle trends, symptoms and the lifestyle. Gloe et al. (2023) have warned, though, that the applicability to clinical use could be limited by algorithmic errors and self-reported data. Nevertheless, digital solutions increase menstrual literacy and prevent early diagnosis of abnormalities. Vollmar et al. (2025) proposed that wearable sensor data combined with a menstrual tracking system should be used to generate a full reproductive health profile. This kind of integration gets us past the subjective and objective physiological measurement.

Menstrual health changes during adolescence to the stage of perimenopause. Cunningham et al. (2024) also reported a rise in variability in the length of the cycle and the severity of symptoms in old age. The study by Xing et al. (2023) also associated the early menstrual termination with the death risk, stating that the menstrual lifespan is the indicator of the overall health. Wang et al. (2023) also linked depressive symptoms to shorter reproductive duration, which is the interdependence of the menstrual health and the mental one.

3.4 COMPUTATIONAL AI-BASED MODELS IN WOMEN'S REPRODUCTIVE MENSTRUAL, AND MENOPAUSAL HEALTH

Reproductive physiology of women is cyclical and dynamic and is marked by hormonal fluctuation over time, inter-individual differences and age-related changes like perimenopause and menopause. As Cunningham et al. (2024) underscored, longitudinal reproductive data are nonlinearly correlated, thus making it difficult to use traditional regression methods. In their turn, ML models are able to detect the hidden patterns of large, heterogeneous data. There is even more complexity added by nutrition. The nutritional consumption interacts with hormonal control, metabolic well-being and flammation pathways, which affect menstrual routine and menopausal symptomology. Benayoun et al. (2025) emphasized that multilayered molecular alterations are essential aspects of reproductive aging that are impossible to properly model without the omics and clinical data as well as lifestyle data and computational models.

ML algorithms with supervision like Logistic Regression, Support Vector Machines (SVM), Random Forests and Gradient Boosting have been applied extensively in reproductive health prediction tasks. These techniques come in handy especially when trying to classify menstrual diseases, anticipate abnormalities of the cycle, and determining predisposing factors of endocrine abnormality. Wang et al. (2022) used the long-term menstrual data and implemented ML models to predict cardiovascular disease risk, and they showed that it outperforms the traditional models. Their results support the idea of the menstrual health as a systemic biomarker, and they explain the potential of ML to reveal clinically significant associations. Random Forest models have demonstrated good results in noisy dealing with menstrual tracking data since they are resistant to overfitting. As it was mentioned by Gloe et al. (2023), ensemble methods are more effective at using self-reported cycle data, which are frequently incomplete or inconsistent.

Convolutional Neural Networks (CNNs), Recurrent Neural Networks (RNNs), and Long Short-Term Memory (LSTM) networks can be used as deep learning architectures to improve menstrual cycle modeling by incorporating a temporal dependency. Particularly, LSTM models are suitable to cycle prediction due to the information that is carried on several time steps. As suggested by Vollmar et al. (2025), wearable sensor data including heart rate variability, skin temperature and sleep duration could be incorporated into deep learning frameworks to improve prediction of cycle phases. Physiological indicators of hormonal states can be more accurately associated using such multimodal approaches. Medical image analysis CNN-based models have also found application in reproductive health medical image analysis (ovarian imaging and endometrial assessment).

Menopause is a major shift characterized by the falling level of estrogen, irregular menstrual periods, and the susceptibility to metabolic and mental illnesses. The occurrence and the development of menopause have been a significant clinical challenge to predict. Xing et al. (2023) showed that early menopause correlates with increased risk of mortality, and indicated the importance of a high-risk detection of women at a young age. Xu et al. (2025) tackled this problem by creating Ovarian aging clock (OvaRePred) which is an AI-based system that combines hormonal and clinical history data as well as molecular data to predict the reproductive aging trajectories. These models are better on predicting than the traditional age-based predictors because they consider inter-individual variations. Wang et al. (2023) also attributed the shorter lifespan of reproductive cycles to more depressive symptoms, and AI-assisted prediction of menopause may allow addressing mental health issues proactively.

Nutrition is becoming a determinant of reproductive health which can be modifiable in computational models. Eating habits affect the metabolism of estrogens, insulin sensitivity, inflammation, and composition of intestinal microbes-all of which affect menstrual and menopausal results. Nagata et al. (2023) emphasized food insecurity as a cause to interfere with menstrual regularity and mental health. The AI models that combine the data on dietary intakes with the hormonal profiles might be used to identify high-risk individuals and propose the individual nutrition interventions. Christanti and Syafiq (2023) also showed that plant-based diets did affect age at menarche, which has long-term implications on reproductive outcomes due to early nutrition in the first years at age. Expanding on the method, AI-based recommender systems can have a more personalized approach to dietary recommendations throughout the reproductive lifespan, especially during perimenopause when nutritional requirements evolve dramatically. Benayoun et al. (2025) noted that the use of anti-inflammatory diets was important in alleviating ovarian aging. The presence of nutrient density scores, intake of micronutrients, and metabolic biomarkers in machine learning models provides a potential pathway in achieving the management of the symptoms of menopause.

Reproductive health is closely connected with psychological well-being especially in menstruation and menopause periods. Schweizer-Schubert et al. (2025) showed neuroendocrine hypersensitivity to hormonal changes makes one susceptible to mood disorders. The application of AI-based stress models based on wearable information and self-reported mood scores can help to detect the state of dysregulation early. Zuo et al. (2025) demonstrated that predictive analytics have a great potential in mental health screening with reproductive history being a significant determinant of postmenopausal depression.

Even with this promise, AI applications in women health have a number of challenges. The issue of data bias is also critical, as most of the datasets do not represent low-income groups and women of older age. Gloe et al. (2023) warned that menstrual tracking apps could usually gather incomplete or commercially biased data, which could not be generalized. The issue of privacy and data security is especially relevant since reproductive health is a sensitive topic. The design of the model, explainable AI, and ethical data management are all critical to build trust and clinical adoption.

3.5 RESEARCH GAP

Although the reproductive health of females had made significant steps in the understanding prevent successful monitoring, prediction and management of menstrual and menopausal health throughout the lifespan. First, although many studies have been done to investigate the biological fundamentals of puberty, menstrual cycles and reproductive aging, most studies are not comprehensive but concentrate on specific parts namely hormonal variations, age of menarche or menstrual abnormalities. Extensive physiological, nutritional and psychosocial measures are not integrated comprehensively, and this limits the capacity to make accurate predictions of reproductive outcomes. Moreover, most of the studies are cross-sectional and they do not provide longitudinal trends in menstrual health, nutrient consumption and psychosocial factors that are critical in analyzing variability over time and different life courses.

Despite the critical importance of nutrition in menstrual regularity, reproductive longevity and the management of menopausal symptoms, recent studies tend to study the effects of specific foods or nutrients individually; instead of using holistic models to account the complex nature of dietary habits, lifestyle practices and socio-economic influences. Accordingly, the delicate diet-menstrual disorders-long-term reproductive health outcomes nexus has not been adequately defined. Equally, psychosocial elements, such as stress, stigma, and hygiene behaviors, have also been identified as providing a significant contribution but are seldom combined with physiological or nutritional information in predictive or intervention-oriented research.

The application of computational and AI-based approaches in women reproductive health is new, but underused. Current models are inclined to predict the menstrual cycle, track the symptoms, or manage menopause separately with little consideration of multi-modal datasets, including nutrition, lifestyle, mental health, and physiological monitoring. The explainable AI models lacking actionable insights to providers and end-users also limit their usage in clinical and personal health settings. Moreover, majority of AI and machine learning models are tested and trained on small populations, which is not always generalizable to the wider demographic, geographic and socio-economic populations.

The translational gap concerning the application of AI-based predictive models and practical nutritional interventions and personalized health recommendations is significantly wide. Although there is evidence that AI is potentially useful in real-time monitoring and predicting symptoms, there are scanty studies that offer evidence-based frameworks to incorporate such predictions into practical dietary or lifestyle changes to adolescent, reproductive-age, or menopausal women. Moreover, current health technologies, such as femtech apps and chatbots, have poor integration of evidence-based culturally sensitive nutritional education, which is essential to make them applicable globally.

Those gaps need an interdisciplinary solution, a combination of biological knowledge, nutritional research, psychosocial knowledge, and AI-based computational solutions. There exists an urgent requirement in longitudinal, population representative studies that make use of multi-modal data to come up with predictive models that could provide individualized, accurate and extremely practical and actionable intervention to reproductive, menstrual and menopausal health of women. Below table 3.1 over view of the previous research.

Table 3.1 Overview of the Previous Research

S.No	Objective	Summary	References
1	To develop an ovarian aging prediction model	The goal of this project was to develop the OvaRePred ovarian ageing clock, a prediction model based on machine learning that calculates reproductive longevity and ovarian ageing. It provides individualized fertility assessments and early warning for reproductive decline by integrating hormonal, genetic, and clinical factors. The approach enhances the decision-making process for fertility interventions and family planning.	Ganguly et al. (2025)
2	To provide comprehensive knowledge in reproductive endocrinology and infertility	Operates as a reliable textbook on topics such as ovarian and uterine physiology, hormone regulation, the causes of infertility, assisted reproductive technologies, and clinical management techniques. It integrates clinical applications for reproductive specialists, gynecologists, and endocrinologists with theoretical underpinnings.	Panjwani et al. (2025)
3	Design a transformer-based menstrual health chatbot	Developed "Mai," a transformer chatbot utilizing NLP for menstrual monitoring, symptom analysis, education, and tailored health suggestions. The chatbot leverages AI to	Hiremath et al. (2025)

		analyses user inputs and deliver precise information about reproductive health, improving accessibility and engagement.	
4	Explore psycho neuroendocrine health using AI	Examines how AI can be used to model psycho-neuroendocrine connections. The study highlights AI's potential in personalized wellness and health monitoring by integrating hormonal, psychological, and physiological data to evaluate mental and reproductive health outcomes.	Omokhabi et al. (2025)
5	Assess menstrual cycle as a vital health indicator	Highlights the significance of menstrual cycle patterns as an essential indicator of general health. The research highlights predictive algorithms for detecting anomalies, linking menstrual health with metabolic, reproductive, and cardiovascular outcomes.	Hemanth et al. (2025)
6	To evaluate femtech applications in reproductive health	Examines mobile applications for menstruation and reproductive tracking in India, emphasising data gathering, measurement of reproductive physiological indicators, and digital interaction. Emphasises the problems related to accuracy, privacy, and socio-cultural acceptance of femtech solutions.	Singh (2025)
7	To study the impact of birth intervals on postmenopausal depression	Examines the relationship between inter-birth intervals and depressed symptoms in postmenopausal women. The research combines epidemiology data and statistical modelling to elucidate the long-term effects of reproductive health on mental well-being.	Kharb & Joshi (2023)

8	Ovarian aging mechanisms	Provides insights into molecular and cellular mechanisms of ovarian aging, including gene expression, DNA damage, and hormonal shifts. Utilizes multi-omics approaches and longitudinal analyses to understand reproductive senescence.	Haq & Khanday (2025)
9	Explore reproductive lifespan and pregnancy loss	Investigates correlations among reproductive lifespan, ovulatory cycles, and miscarriage chances. Employs cohort studies and statistical modelling to elucidate clinical therapies for fertility preservation.	Redman (2024)
10	To examine premature menopause and mortality	Evaluates the association between early menopause and long-term mortality risk. Employs population-based datasets to associate hormonal decline with cardiovascular, metabolic, and neurological consequences.	Adeleye & Zamah (2023)
11	Analyze precision nutrition for menopause cardiovascular risk	Evaluates dietary interventions utilising nutrigenomics to mitigate cardiovascular risk in menopausal women. Emphasises the integration of macronutrient optimization, micronutrient supplementation, and lifestyle modifications.	Mughal et al. (2025)
12	Predict progesterone–estradiol ratio using explainable ML	Enhances knowledge of endocrine dynamics and promotes open clinical decision-making by using explainable machine learning to estimate hormone ratios throughout the menstrual cycle.	Oliveira et al. (2024)
13	To study mechanisms of menstrual and non-	Examines the pathophysiology of migraine during monthly and non-menstrual phases, incorporating hormonal variations, neurovascular mechanisms, and	Wang et al. (2022)

	menstrual migraines	symptomatology to enhance therapy techniques.	
14	Conduct a digital cohort study in PCOS	Establishes a digital health cohort for PCOS patients to monitor symptoms, biochemical indicators, and lifestyle modifications utilising AI-driven analytics. Offers insights for early identification and tailored management.	Kim et al. (2022)
15	To explore reproductive duration and depression	Examines the relationship between women's depressive symptoms and their reproductive span (from menarche to menopause). uses longitudinal research to determine the psychological and hormonal components of mental health.	Kusters et al. (2021)
16	Interpret reproductive hormones across puberty	Offers directives for the clinical assessment of hormone levels during puberty, focussing on normative ranges, pathogenic variations, and diagnostic factors in teenage females.	Wright (2021)
17	To examine hormonal influences on women's respiratory health	Examines the relationship between sex hormones and respiratory diseases, including as COPD and asthma, emphasising immune-endocrine processes that influence the development and course of these ailments.	Zhang et al. (2023)
18	To analyze nutrient-dense food intake across the life course	Assesses the influence of nutrition on female reproductive health, metabolic parameters, and age-associated hormonal alterations. Highlights the significance of micronutrients, the equilibrium of macronutrients, and enduring dietary approaches.	Figueiredo et al. (2024)

19	Assess thyroid dysfunction in women	Investigates the prevalence, aetiology, and reproductive consequences of thyroid problems in Korean women, encompassing impacts on the menstrual cycle, fertility, and metabolic health.	Sen et al. (2024)
20	Analyze menopausal age and Parkinson's disease risk	Examines the correlation between menopausal age and the risk of Parkinson's disease. Emphasises hormonal factors in neurodegeneration and prospective preventative measures.	Cabre et al. (2024)
21	To explore intelligence, puberty, and reproductive outcomes	Analyses cognitive capacity, onset of puberty, and reproductive behaviors, synthesizing evolutionary, physiological, and statistical frameworks to elucidate the factors of reproductive success.	Hansen et al. (2025)
22	Analyze menstrual cycles in non-human primates	Performs a comparative analysis of composite menstrual cycles in captive orangutans, utilising hormonal, behavioural, and cycle monitoring data to enhance research in evolutionary and reproductive biology.	Durgavich et al. (2023)

3.6 SUMMARY

Chapter 3 concentrates on the prompt detection of coffee plant illnesses, which is essential for diagnosing and alleviating the considerable difficulties these conditions provide. As a result, the current study employed AI-driven recommendation systems LSTM, Red Fox Optimisation (RFO), Explainable Artificial Intelligence (XAI), Agri-IoT, DFNET, and DCNN. Prior research has demonstrated that AI-driven Machine Vision techniques are effective for the prompt detection of coffee plant illnesses, necessitating no prior training. As a result, a number of earlier research projects have incorporated artificial intelligence (AI) powered machine vision algorithms since they are better at accurately forecasting coffee plant diseases.

CHAPTER 4

AN INTELLIGENT MACHINE LEARNING-BASED PERSONALIZED NUTRITION RECOMMENDATION FOR ADOLESCENT GIRLS AT MENARCHE

4.1 INTRODUCTION

Menarche refers to the first period of menstruation in young girls, and it represents the reproductive maturity. The average age of menarche in the world is 12-13 years old, but it may be as early as 9 years of age and as late as 15 years of age depending on the variables of the genetics, the environment and nutrition. Menarche is a very significant milestone in the female reproductive health, since it is eloquently linked with hormone cycle regulation, the onset of secondary sexual traits and the readiness of the body to conceive. This stage is characterized with significant physiological changes that are affected by hormonal interactions between the hypothalamus, the pituitary gland, and the ovaries, leading to the production of oestrogen and progesterone. Physiological Processes that mediate Menarche: Hypothalamic pituitary gonadal (HPG) axis plays a major role in the initiation of menarche. The gonadotropin-releasing hormone (GnRH) is secreted by the hypothalamus and triggers the synthesis of follicle-stimulating hormone (FSH) and luteinizing hormone (LH) by the anterior pituitary. These hormones make the ovaries to secret estrogen and progesterone, therefore, regulating the menstrual cycle and enhancing maturity of the reproductive organs. Menstrual cycle is divided into three stages, which include: follicular, ovulation and luteal stages with hormonal changes in each stage. Nutritional Requirements at Menarche: Menarche nutrition is very important in ensuring the development of the body is rapid, balance of hormones, and the increase in menstruation discomfort is countered. The nutrients, which are necessary to relieve cramps, lethargy, bloating, and mood swings, are iron, folate, calcium, magnesium, omega-3 fatty acids, and vitamin B6. Hemoglobin production and anaemia prevention, Iron and folate are needed; relaxation in muscles, calcium and magnesium; anti-inflammatory effects, omega-3 fatty acids; mood, vitamin B6.

Genetic, environmental, and lifestyle factors: Genetic predisposition markedly influences the timing of menarche, with daughters frequently attaining menarche at an age akin to that of their mothers. Environmental factors, including socioeconomic position, exposure to stress, and endocrine-disrupting substances, can either hasten or postpone the beginning of menarche. The nutritional quality, especially fat consumption, significantly influences oestrogen synthesis and menstrual regularity. Cultural, Psychological, and Health Implications: Cultural interpretations of menarche differ significantly; in certain groups, it is commemorated as a rite of passage into womanhood, whilst in others, it is enveloped in stigma and taboos. Misunderstandings and insufficient education can result in psychological pain, anxiety, and humiliation. From a health perspective, early menarche is associated with elevated risks of breast cancer, obesity, and cardiovascular illnesses, while late menarche may heighten the risk of osteoporosis. Figure 4.1 During menarche, the female reproductive system grows as hormones such as GnRH, FSH, and LH stimulate the ovaries to create oestrogen and progesterone. This results in the uterus forming a denser lining, while the vaginal walls get increased elasticity. The menstrual cycle commences, signifying the body's preparedness for potential reproduction and overall well-being.

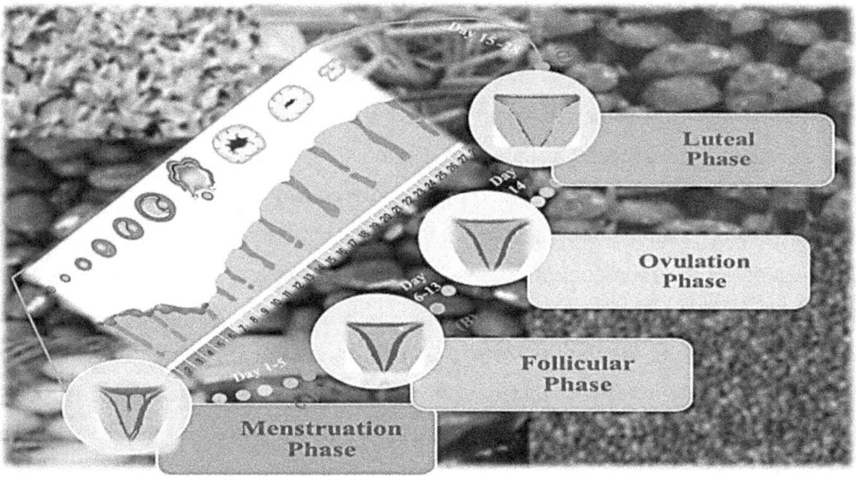

Figure 4.1. Female Reproductive System

4.2 PROPOSED WORK

Using open-access resources and thorough symptom severity records, the project gathers data from teenage girls going through menarche. Concerns about dietary consumption and symptomatology during the first menstrual cycle are first highlighted in the study. The two primary parts of the suggested work framework are data collection and preparation, which includes improved feature selection methods that make it easier to include pertinent qualities into predictive models as well as data cleaning, normalisation, and outlier elimination. By modelling the relationship between dietary intake and the intensity of menstrual symptoms using machine learning algorithms like Rule-based Random Forest, K-Nearest Neighbours (KNN), and eXtreme Gradient Boosting (XGBoost), individualised nutrition recommendations are produced for better menstrual health outcomes. A procedure for advising teenage girls on diet at menarche is shown in figure 4.2. The first step in the process is gathering information from each member of the cohort, including food consumption and symptoms. To guarantee the excellent quality of the data, the raw data is then cleaned, normalised, and any missing values are filled in. Using feature selection, the model's best components are chosen. The prepared data is then fed into Model Training, where predictive models are trained utilising rule-based Random Forest, KNN, and XGBoost machine learning techniques. Model evaluation examines each model's performance by taking into account its accuracy, precision, recall, and F1-score. When a dietary suggestion is produced based on the model predictions the cycle is over.

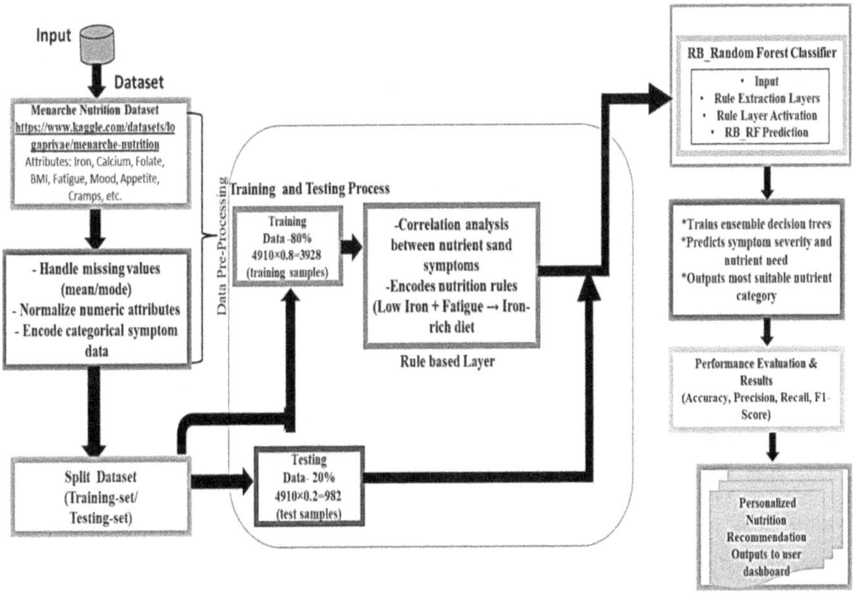

Figure 4.2. Proposed Work for Adolescent Females at Menarche

Nutrition for Women First During Menstruation

Subsequent to menarche, a girl should implement a nutritious diet to regulate hormonal changes, alleviate monthly discomfort, and stabilise mood and energy levels. Iron, calcium, vitamin D, vitamin B12, folic acid, omega-3 fatty acids, and dietary fibre are crucial for individuals with digestive disorders because of their health benefits. Nutrients in tailored diets can aid ladies during the onset of menstruation and improve their well-being. NHANES suggests that dysmenorrhea may lead to menstrual periods that vary from mild to severe, along with back problems, abdominal discomfort, mood swings, and irritability. Nutritional beverages can augment energy levels and mitigate cramps, hence improving women's menstrual health.

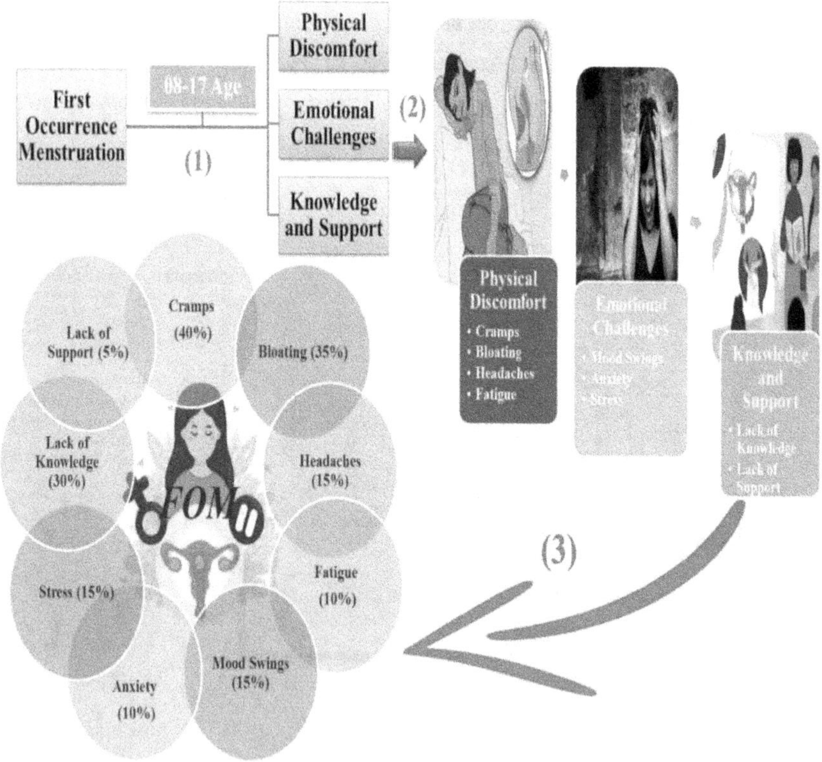

Figure 4.3. Women's first menstrual cycle an important component of resource

The aforementioned figure 4.3 illustrates that a key feature of this resource is its thorough examination of the common challenges women may encounter throughout their initial menstrual cycle. An additional crucial element of this resource is its capacity to furnish information sources. Planned Parenthood, the American Academy of Paediatrics, the National Institutes of Health, and the Mayo Clinic are all highly esteemed organisations. Employing search engines such as Google Scholar and PubMed, the subsequent stage is to obtain publications and surveys relevant to the current situation. This may be achieved through the use of the internet. A professional opinion is expressed concerning the assessment of menstrual cycles and the present condition of women's health.

4.2.1 DATA COLLECTION AND PROCESSING

Data obtained from publicly accessible open datasets regarding menstrual nutrition, including nutritional facts and symptom ranges. Missing data was addressed by imputation approaches utilising both the mean and mode throughout the preprocessing phase. The data features have been standardised to prevent the models from being influenced by scale discrepancies during training. Machine learning models can manage nutritional preferences and dietary groups when encoded using one-hot encoding.

4.3 MACHINE LEARNING ALGORITHM MODEL ARCHITECTURE

Investigating the correlation between nutrition and severe menstruation symptoms with machine learning methodologies, including Rule-based Random Forest, K-Nearest Neighbours (KNN), and eXtreme Gradient Boosting (XGBoost). An impartial assessment in performance evaluation necessitates a data-segregating training pipeline for utilisation during both training and testing phases. Rule-based Random Forest effectively manages intricate and nonlinear interactions among data, making it suitable for feature ranking and exploratory modelling. Although XGBoost utilises gradient boosting to predict meal accuracy, KNN is employed to determine specific nutritional content across diverse domains.

Standardization of Nutrient

$$P_{std} = \frac{P - \mu}{\sigma} \tag{4.1}$$

This equation advises appropriate nutrition during menarche using common information for all its measures and by standardizing the nutrition data by obtaining the μ and σ values.

Missing Value Imputation Using KNN

$$\hat{P}_l = \frac{1}{s}\sum_{j=1}^{s} P_j \tag{4.2}$$

This updates the mean consumption from S similar individuals. This guarantees that the AI model possesses precise data to suggest iron-rich diets to alleviate menarche-associated cramps and weariness.

Z-score for Outlier Detection

$$Z = \frac{P - \beta}{\sigma} \tag{4.3}$$

Z-scores are used to identify these outliers. Values of Z above or below a threshold guarantee appropriate nutritional suggestions that specifically addresses the symptoms of the first menstruation.

Significance Score for Random Forest Functions

$$FS_l = \frac{1}{n}\sum_{t=1}^{n} \Delta Gini_t \tag{4.4}$$

Rather than classification accuracy to, Gini impurity from the Rule based Random Forest algorithm was analysed for menarche symptoms. It explains the significance of necessary nutrients in supporting healthy menstruation, so it is easier to advise nutritional changes for menstruating teens.

Euclidean Distance in KNN

$$d(x,y) = \sqrt{\sum_{l=1}^{n}(x_l - y_l)^2} \tag{4.5}$$

Using this metric, KNN dietary recommendations are made based on the most similar historical profiles.

A Prediction of Rule based Random Forest

$$\hat{y} = \frac{1}{n}\sum_{l=1}^{n} T_l(x) \tag{4.6}$$

Ensemble prediction is made by combining multiple $Ti(x)$ individual decision trees. The level of symptoms is predicted by the mean output of the model.

KNN Prediction

$$\hat{y} = \frac{1}{k}\sum_{l=1}^{k} y_l \quad (4.7)$$

Calculates the average of the results of the k nearest neighbours. This is critical for determining nutritional recommendations.

Objective Function of XGBoost

$$V(\theta) = \sum_{l=1}^{n} v(y_l, \hat{y}_l) + \sum_{k=1}^{k} \Omega(f_k) \quad (4.8)$$

Work towards fairness between the line in the data $v(y_l, \hat{y}_l)$ to avoid increasing model error include regularisation functions $\Omega(f_k)$ in method. Because of this can use robust nutritional predictions in many different populations.

Pseudocode for Machine Learning Feature Selection

PersonalizedNutritionRecommendation_Menarche

Input: Open_Nutrition_Dataset

Symptom_Severity_Profiles

Output:

Tailored_Nutrition_Recommendations for each adolescent female at menarche

Step 1: Data Acquisition and Preprocessing

-Load Open_Nutrition_Dataset and Symptom_Severity_Profiles

- Merge datasets using unique participant identifiers
- Handle missing values (mean/mode imputation for numerical/categorical data)
- Normalize continuous features to a standard scale
- Encode categorical features

Step 2: Feature Engineering and Selection

- Perform correlation analysis to identify relationships between dietary intake and symptoms

- Use Rule based Random Forest feature importance scores to rank features
- Select top N features to reduce dimensionality and improve model efficiency

Step 3: Model Development

- Split data into training and testing sets (80% training, 20% testing)
- Initialize machine learning models:
- Model_RF ← Rule based Random Forest Classifier
- Model_KNN ← K-Nearest Neighbors Classifier
- Model_XGB ← XGBoost Classifier
- For each model:
- Train model on training set using selected features
- Evaluate using testing set to obtain accuracy, precision, recall, F1-score

Step 4: Model Comparison and Selection

- Compare models based on accuracy and precision metrics
- Select Best_Model ← model with highest accuracy and precision

Step 5: Personalized Nutrition Recommendation Generation

- Input new participant data
- Use Best_Model to predict symptom severity for new participant
- Identify key nutrients linked to alleviating predicted symptoms
- Generate personalized nutrition plan, mapping recommended nutrients to specific dietary sources

Step 6: Output and User Profile Integration

- Display tailored nutrition recommendations to the user
- Store recommendations in user profile for future monitoring and adjustments.

4.3.1 SPECIFICS OF THE DATASET

The Kaggle dataset and the food nutrient open dataset are used in this study. This dataset includes data on food nutrition, including trends in dietary intake as well as macronutrients and micronutrients. The collection includes common menarche-related symptoms in table 4.1.

Table 4.1. Summary of the Dataset Utilised for Nutritional Recommendation

Dataset Attribute	Description
Data Source	Kaggle and open data (Nutrition)
Target Variable	Menarche symptom severity
Nutrients Covered	Iron, calcium, vitamin D, B12, folic acid, omega-3, fiber, etc.
Data Format	CSV, numeric and categorical

Experimental Protocol

The data was divided into 80% training samples and 20% testing samples in table 4.2.

- Data preparation involves managing missing values and applying normalization to data.
- Utilise Rule-based Random Forest, K-Nearest Neighbours, and XGBoost for model training.
- Assessment of performance metrics on test data utilising accuracy, precision, recall, and F1-score.
- The results are more stable due to the implementation of ten-fold cross-validation.

Table 4.2. Parameter Settings

Experimental Step	Details
Train-Test Split	80%: 20%
Preprocessing	Normalization, missing data imputation
Algorithms Used	Rule based Random Forest, KNN, XGBoost
Validation Technique	10-fold cross-validation
Evaluation Metrics	Accuracy, precision, recall, F1-score, execution time

Nutrition Recommendation

$$NR_l = \sum_{j=1}^{n} \omega_j . P_{lj} \qquad (4.9)$$

A numerical value showing the importance of nutritional recommendations. The importance of nutrients to menarche symptoms decides their weights, so a suitable nutrition plan is created for the patient.

Nutrition Intake Prediction

$$\hat{N} = f(P; \theta) \qquad (4.10)$$

The model delivers its prediction of what a person should take every day P. The recommend given works best for those who are new to menstruation.

Error Term

$$\epsilon = y - \hat{y} \qquad (4.11)$$

The challenge in forecasting results. This discrepancy can be mitigated by using the AI to tailor nutrition programs according to the symptoms experienced by menstruation.

Symptom Severity Prediction

$$S = \beta_0 + \sum_{l=1}^{h} \beta_l P_l \qquad (4.12)$$

It expresses symptom severity (S) by summing up the nutrients involved.

Model Loss Function

$$L = \frac{1}{n} \sum_{l=1}^{n} (y_l - \hat{y}_l)^2 \qquad (4.13)$$

Stands in contrast the model nutritional recommendations with the observed alterations in symptoms. A low loss indicates that nutritional selections are beneficial for menarche health.

Nutrition Relevance

$$NRS = \frac{Nutrition_l}{Total\ Nutrition} \qquad (4.14)$$

Nutrients play a part in diet and they help ease early menstruation symptoms which commonly include anemia and exhaustion.

4.4 SUMMARY

This study combines symptom-based and nutritional feature modelling to develop a machine learning-driven personalised nutrition advice system for adolescent females during menarche. The system improves nutrition planning by correlating menstrual symptom severity with nutrient intake through thorough preprocessing, feature selection, and multi-algorithm modelling. The system assesses three machine learning methodologies: Rule-based Random Forest, K-Nearest Neighbours (KNN), and XGBoost, to determine the most efficacious predictive model. Experimental results indicate that the Rule-based Random Forest algorithm attains superior performance, achieving 92% accuracy in symptom prediction and 89% precision in food prescription, surpassing other models. The assessment of accuracy, precision, recall, and F1-score validates the robustness of the suggested system. The results underscore the promise of integrating targeted nutritional research with sophisticated AI algorithms to enhance menstrual health management. The use of open-access datasets, symptom-oriented feature engineering, and comparison model analysis signifies a substantial progression in the creation of personalised healthcare solutions.

CHAPTER 5

HYBRID GREYLAG GOOSE WITH LAYERED SPARSE NETWORK FOR WOMEN NUTRITION SUGGESTIONS DURING MENSTRUAL CYCLE

5.1 INTRODUCTION

In human beings and primates, the most noticeable aspect of the menstrual cycle is the periodic bleeding of the vagina caused by the shedding of uterine mucosa which is called menstruation. At the female reproductive system this can be seen as a cyclic preparation process to fertilisation and gestation. Female reproductive system experiences normal cyclical changes. Although it is notorious with its unpredictability, the average menstrual cycle period is 28 days since the start of one menstrual cycle up to the initiation of the next one. The first day of the cycle is not only when the day count of the cycle begins as popularly believed but it is also on the first day of the menstrual period. It begins with puberty which happens between age 10 and 16 and usually ends at the menopause age which is 51. During the menstrual period, the women would often experience mood swings, craving foods, stomach cramps, bloating as well as headaches. These symptoms are more or less severe depending on hormonal changes at follicular, menstrual, luteal and ovulatory phases. When unattended, the above symptoms could have negative impacts on health and day to day operations.

A growing body of research recommends the use of nutrition to ensure good health and control these symptoms during the menstrual period. Some of the key nutrients that are essential to minimise the severity of the symptoms, ensure hormonal balance, and lead to greater vitality are calcium, magnesium, iron, and vitamin D. In recent years, various approaches have been used to make individualised recommendations. However, the lack of individualised, data-driven nutrition plans that are responsive to specific needs of women in various stages of their life does not exist. The primary concern is the sole use of collaborative or content-based methods of filters, which may result in a downstream of suggestions. Collaborative filtering may become a problem when the new items or users have little or no data on which to base more efficient recommendations, a phenomenon known as the cold start problem, since the content-based algorithms have not considered the varied experiences and interests of dissimilar users. Also, most of the systems fail to take into account physiological and psychological changes that occur in women during their menstrual periods that leads to some suggestions that do not take into consideration specific symptoms or nutritional requirements.

Machine learning (ML) is considered a branch of Artificial Intelligence (AI) which allows systems to learn concepts and information through autonomous (i.e. not explicitly programmed) means. The traditional machine learning methods include random forests (RF), Naive Bayes (NB), support vectors machines (SVM) and K-nearest neighbours (KNN) which can be applied in various projects such as cancer detection, pest identification, and dietary prediction. The prediction of PCOS entails the use of a web-based machine learning framework that assists in the early detection. The maximum accuracy level that has been attained by this method is 94%. A RF based on knowledge graphs is used to forecast both environmental and nutritional factors related to the female reproductive problem, with higher results. However, the prevailing machine learning models continued to rely on manual feature extraction to train models.

In turn, over the last ten years, an increasing number of studies use deep learning (DL) algorithms, which provide the automatic extraction of features and are more accurate than the old-fashioned machine learning (ML) applications. The deep learning methods, such as deep belief networks (DBN), convolutional neural networks (CNN), and ResNet, have proven to make considerable progress in a wide range of applications, which point to impressive performance and offer desirable functionalities. Osprey Gannet optimisation is used to illustrate the use of CNN-based transfer learning to predict cardiovascular risk on retinal fundus pictures. To accomplish this, a sophisticated deep learning model has been created to estimate the level of nutrient present in soil to grow cabbage.

A cardiovascular disease prediction deep residual network employing a chronological chef-based optimisation has been put forward, with the highest accuracy of 89.8. In addition, autonomous food recognition has been done using deep convolutional neural networks with self-attention processes. The model demonstrated a very high level of accuracy with 95.11 on the MA Food-121 dataset and 96.40 on the Food-101 dataset. In the framework of women nutrition guidelines, DL has the opportunity to revolutionise women healthcare delivery with the opportunity to offer personalised nutritional advice guided by individualised health information and real-time symptom update. However, the most popular deep learning models can be affected by overfitting issues and they do not model complex interactions sufficiently. The present study presents a new hybrid deep learning model that will consider numerous variables, among which are the menstruation phases, symptoms, and personal health history, and will help to make individual dietary suggestions. The methodology will address the gaps in the nutritional counsel, which is often not personalised, and does not take into consideration the dynamic nature of the women health throughout the menstrual cycles. The model uses a combined deep learning approach, which uses a combination of different neural network designs to identify complex patterns in data. Hyper-parameter values are tuned to optimise model classification and reduce overfitting and achieve an efficient model training. The effectiveness of the model is measured in various ways to illustrate its effectiveness as compared to the existing methodologies. Furthermore, it will be aimed at empowering women to actively take control of their health and pay in the growing sphere of tailor-made nutrition and health provision. With this holistic treatment, the existing nutritional needs are addressed, and how to achieve a more comprehensive insight into the connection between menstruation health and diet is nurtured.

5.2 PROPOSED METHODOLOGY

This part is about another new model of OdriHDL model that aims at proposing nutritional wellness to women during their menstrual cycle. The main goal of the suggested OdriHDL model is to examine complex patterns and give specific, individual recommendations, which will enhance menstrual health and well-being. The first stage is the pre-processing phase where the input data is first processed and that includes mood swings, headaches, bloating, fatigue, acne, breast tenderness, cramps, and the personal health data e.g. the level of stress, BMI, and age. This data is polished with the help of Missing Value Imputation, Z-score Normalisation, and One-hot Encoding. Afterward, extracting features is done with the help of Layered Sparse Autoencoder Network (LSAENet) to find the important features that explain the relationship between nutritional needs and menstruation symptoms. After that, a nutrient recommendation is implemented using the obtained characteristics with the Hybrid Attention-based Bidirectional Convolutional Greylag Goose Gated Recurrent Network (HABi-ConGRNet). To enhance the rate of classification performance, the Greylag Goose Optimisation Algorithm (GGOA) is used to optimise the hyper-parameter of the classification model. The suggested method classifies the nutrient levels (e.g. magnesium, iron, calcium and vitamin D) as moderate, low and high.

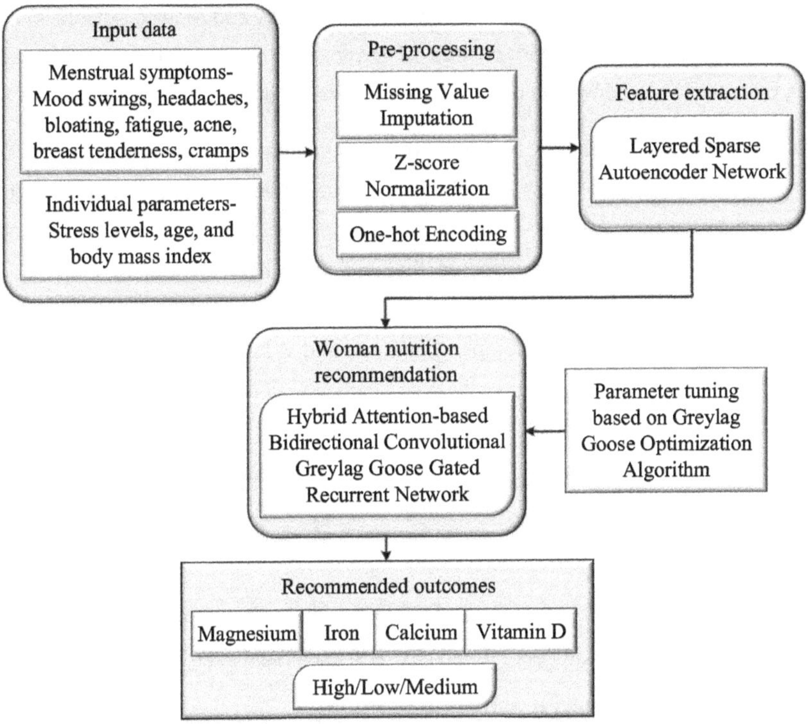

Figure 5.1. Block diagram of OdriHDL model

Figure 5.1 illustrates the block diagram of the OdriHDL model, showcasing the data flow through various stages including pre-processing, feature extraction, and nutritional guidance. This design adeptly identifies intricate patterns in input data concerning women's nutritional needs during the menstrual cycle. Integrating these steps enhances data quality, extracts significant features, and elevates the model's overall efficacy in delivering tailored recommendations.

5.2.1 DATA PRE-PROCESSING

Data pre-processing is essential for creating a reliable and stable system before implementing deep learning algorithms in the model. A sequence of data pre-processing procedures is performed to ensure the dataset is sanitised and prepared for model training. The proposed study has recognised absent values in dietary recommendations for women's health during the menstrual cycle and utilised a data imputation technique to rectify these deficiencies.

Z-score normalisation techniques have been utilised to identify and replace outliers. Categorical variables, such as symptoms and phases of the menstrual cycle (e.g., menstrual, luteal, follicular, ovulation), are converted into numerical values by one-hot encoding.

Missing value imputation: For the purpose of imputation of missing data, the proposed method uses k-nearest neighbours (KNN). kNN imputes missing data by using the distance between sample vectors in the dataset's space. For every missing feature, it calculates the average values of the k nearest samples that use the observed feature in connection to numerical data. The outcome for categorical data is represented by the KNN algorithm's prevalent class. Given a sample $s(x,y,0)$ and its k nearest neighbors $N_k = \{\{x_j, y_j, 1) \mid j = 1,2,...,k\}$, we define:

$$y = \begin{cases} \arg\max_Z \left\{ \sum_{(x_j y_j, 1) \in N_k} 1(y_j = Z) \right\} & \textit{if y is categorical} \\ \frac{1}{5} \sum_{j=1}^{k} y_j & \textit{if y is numerical} \end{cases} \tag{5.1}$$

As there are only binary values, Z can only be either 1 or 0, and $1(y_j = Z)$ resembles a function that returns 0 when $(y_j = Z)$ and else returns 0. The euclidean is the metric utilized to compute the distance between two points q and r:

$$D(q,r) = \sum_{j=1}^{p} (r_j - q_j)^2 \tag{5.2}$$

where, p describes how many variables there are for all of the data points.

Z-score normalization: Before implementing any models, it is essential to normalise numerical features, as scaling is requisite for numerous techniques, including deep learning. This proposed method employs Z-score normalisation, commonly referred to as zero-mean normalisation, among many scaling strategies. The mean and standard deviation are employed to standardise the values of a characteristic. The formula for Z-score normalisation can be expressed as:

$$Z = \frac{y - v}{\chi} \tag{5.3}$$

where, Z indicates the Z-score value, y signifies the feature value, v represents the mean value and χ states the standard deviation.

One-hot Encoding: The conversion of non-numerical features, such as categorical values, into numerical values is required by the models in order to enhance the efficiency of model training. To convert the categorical features into n-dimensional binary code vectors, where n represents the total number of attributes in the category feature, one-hot-encoding technique is employed.

5.2.2 LAYERED SPARSE AUTOENCODER NETWORK

Feature extraction is a procedure that involves detecting and extracting significant information that aid in recommending nutritional wellness for women during their menstrual cycle. An autoencoder (AE) is a neural network architecture designed to learn latent features (compressed representations) of data by recreating the input data at the output stage. It consists of two components: an encoder that transforms the input into latent space, and a decoder that seeks patterns within the lower-dimensional latent space. A sparse autoencoder improves the efficiency of important feature extraction by enforcing sparsity on the hidden units. In the proposed OdriHDL model, feature extraction is conducted using a Layered Sparse Autoencoder Network (LSAENet) to identify relevant characteristics that elucidate the link between dietary requirements and menstruation symptoms. A neural network consisting of multiple sparse autoencoders connected end-to-end is referred to as an LSAENet. To obtain high-level feature representations of the input data, the output from the preceding layer of the sparse self-encoder is transmitted to the following layer of the self-encoder. Figure 5.2 depicts the architecture of the LSAENet neural network for feature extraction. The output of each layer functions as the input for the subsequent layer. This facilitates the derivation of advanced feature representations from the input data. The LSAENet layers are trained progressively using the greedy layer-wise pre-training method to achieve optimal connection weights and bias values for the entire sparse AE network layers.

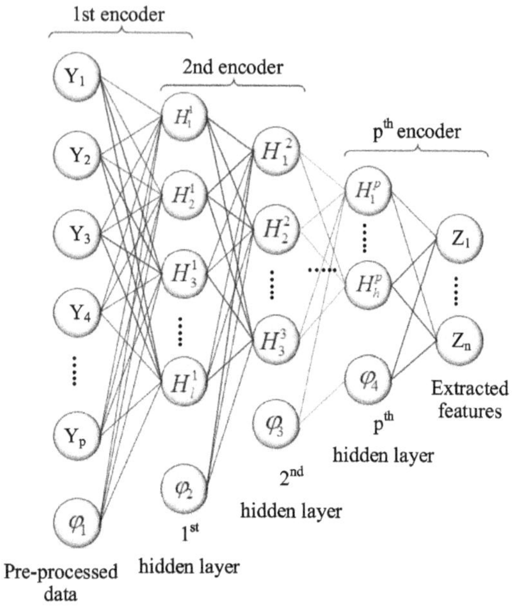

Figure 5.2. Structure of LSAENet

Then, to acquire the best parameter model, the LSAENet is fine-tuned by means of an error back propagation approach until the error function results between the output and input data meets the expected requirements.

For error function $K_{sparse}(\omega, bi)$:

$$\frac{\partial}{\partial \omega_{jk}^{s}} K_{sparse}(\omega, bi) = \frac{1}{2p_s} \sum_{s=1}^{p_s} K_{sparse}(\omega, bi, Y(p), Z(p)) + \kappa \omega_{jk}^{s} \tag{5.4}$$

$$\frac{\partial}{\partial bi^{s}} K_{sparse}(\omega, bi) = \frac{1}{2p_s} \sum_{s=1}^{p_s} \frac{\partial}{\partial bi^{s}} K_{sparse}(\omega, bi, Y(p), Z(p)) \tag{5.5}$$

Thereby, the weight and bias update process is given as follows:

$$\omega_{jk}^{l} = \omega_{jk}^{l} - \mu \frac{\partial}{\partial \omega_{jk}^{l}} K(\omega, bi) \tag{5.6}$$

$$bi^s = bi^s - \mu \frac{\partial}{\partial bi^s} K(\omega, bi) \quad (5.7)$$

where, ω indicates the weight connection between AE layers, bi resembles the bias associated with neurons in AE, μ resembles the update learning rate, $Y(p)$ and $Z(p)$ resembles the pth original vector and its resultant reconstruction vector. Besides, ω_{jk}^{l} designates the weight connecting j^{th} neuron preceding layer to k^{th} neuron of present layer in l^{th} layer of LSAENet, p_s indicates the output of sth neuron, and bi^s signifies the bias associated with s^{th} neuron in the neural network layer.

The various parameters have different learning rates, such as reduce the rate of update of uncommon features, as the LSAENet network has sparse restrictions. However, most popular standard gradient descent methods, including the mini-batch gradient descent and stochastic gradient descent, use the same learning rate in all the parameters of the network in need of learning. It becomes hard to select a suitable learning rate and rapidly affect at local minimum. As a result, an adaptive moment estimation (Adam) gradient descent method is applied to realize dynamic adaptive modification of other parameters to train LSAENet. By computing the gradient 1st order moment estimate n_u and 2nd -order moment estimate V_u, as indicated in formula (8-10), the Adam algorithm allows for the dynamic adjustment of various parameters. Here, δ_1 and δ_2 represent the first- and second-order exponential damping decrements, respectively. The parameters gradient at timestep u in the loss function $K_{sparse}(\omega, bi)$ is signified by h_u.

$$n_u = \delta_1 n_{u-1} + (1-\delta_1).h_u \quad (5.8)$$

$$V_u = \delta_2 V_{u-1} + (1-\delta_2).h_u^2 \quad (5.9)$$

$$h_u \leftarrow \nabla_\varphi K_u(\varphi_{u-1}) \quad (5.10)$$

where, ∇_φ indicates the gradient operation corresponding to the parameter φ, K_u implies the gradient of loss, $K_u(\varphi_{u-1})$ specifies the error function computed at parameter (weight or bias) φ from the preceding iteration $u-1$.

The bias corrected for n_u and V_u can be given as:

$$n_u^{'} = \frac{n_u}{1-\delta_1^u} \tag{5.11}$$

$$V_u^{'} = \frac{V_u}{1-\delta_2^u} \tag{5.12}$$

Update parameters:

$$\varphi_{u+1} = \varphi_u - \frac{\zeta}{\sqrt{V_u^{'}} + \psi} . n_u^{'} \tag{5.13}$$

where, ζ represents the update stepsize, and ψ indicates a small constant to avoid the denominator to be 0.

5.2.3 HYBRID ATTENTION-BASED BIDIRECTIONAL CONVOLUTIONAL GREYLAG GOOSE GATED RECURRENT NETWORK

Following feature extraction, the proposed OdriHDL model utilises a Hybrid Attention-based Bidirectional Convolutional Greylag Goose Gated Recurrent Network (HABi-ConGRNet) for nutritional recommendations for women's health during the menstrual cycle. HABi-ConGRNet integrates Convolutional Neural Networks (CNN), bidirectional Gated Recurrent Units (BiGRU), a cross-attention mechanism (CrAM), and the Greylag Goose Optimisation Algorithm (GGOA). The CNN obtains geographic correlations between health measurements and nutrients following feature extraction, which detects essential variables such as age, cycle stages, and health problems. It identifies patterns in dietary needs, such as the increased demand for iron during menstruation or calcium during the luteal phase. The BiGRU addresses the sequential nature of the menstrual cycle by acquiring knowledge of the time-dependent variations in nutritional requirements throughout different phases. BiGRU aids in forecasting the most critical nutrients at specific phases of the cycle by recognising these fluctuations. Consequently, the CrAM dynamically allocates a higher priority to certain aspects, such as iron during menstruation and magnesium during other stages, among others. This guarantees that recommendations are closely aligned with the present stage and condition. By integrating both methodologies, the hybrid model adeptly discerns both cyclical patterns and specific nutritional priorities to provide tailored health nutrition advice that adapts to the evolving needs of users throughout the menstrual cycle.

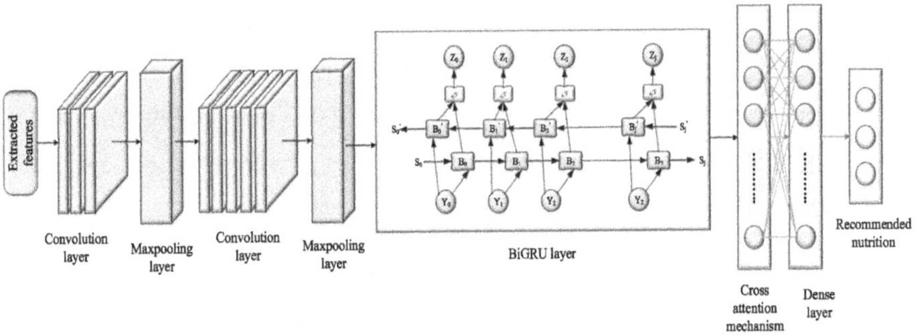

Figure 5.3. Architecture of HABi-ConGRNet model

The architecture of the HABi-ConGRNet model is shown in Figure 5.3. It reflects the progressive order of features in most of the parts such as the input layer, several convolutional layers, max pooling layer and BiGRU layer, an element that represents time dependencies in the data. Moreover, a cross-attention mechanism (CrAM) is incorporated in order to highlight important details. It will allow the program to change the dietary advice according to the specific stage of a menstrual cycle and personal health parameters.

Convolutional neural network

CNN is regarded as one of the representative algorithms of DL. It is a deep-structured feedforward neural network, which involves convolution computation. The system of biological visual perception was adopted in the development of CNN. The paucity of connecting links between layers and sharing of convolution kernel parameter of the hidden layer enables the CNN to extract features at minimum computation. The whole structure of CNN is the input layer, convolutional layer, pooling layer and fully connected (FC) layer. The extracted features are inputted in input layer. The convolutional layer performs convolutional computation with the input using convolutional kernel to obtain feature map. In most cases, multiple convolution kernels are used to carry out the feature extraction process in order to harness the convolution kernels to a greater advantage. The combination encompassing Z convolution kernels is signified by $[Q_1, Q_2, Q_3, \ldots, Q_Z]$, where Q_Z resembles Z^{th} convolution kernel size, or the convolution kernel window's longitudinal dimension. The vector dimension of feature vector is equal to the horizontal convolution kernel window size.

There will be Z feature map vectors after calculating Z convolution kernels. The convolution window size is given as I. The convolution kernel is applied to carry out the convolution operation on the input windows $y_1^H, y_2^H, y_3^H, ..., y_{p-H+1}^p$ to extract the local features. Assume that the input D comprises of p feature vectors, $y_1, y_2, y_3, ..., y_p$, the convolutional layer's function can be written as:

$$z_j = g(X.y_{j:j+H-1} + B) \tag{5.14}$$

where, $g(*)$ signifies the nonlinear function, H resembles the dimension of the convolution kernel, B specifies the bias vector and X indicates the weight matrix. The combination of vectors is represented by the symbol $y_{j:j+H-1}$.

After the extraction of the convolution kernel, the eigenvector z is obtained as:

$$z = \{z_1, z_2, z_3, ..., z_{p-H+1}\} \tag{5.15}$$

Following the convolution operation, each eigenvector is exposed to pooling processing by means of the pooling layer. The multidimensional vector is transformed into a value after pooling, which is utilized as a pooled vector element. The sequence output from convolutional layer is passed into the pooling layer using maximum pooling approach, which is used by the pooling layer. The largest element in the series $z_1, z_2, z_3, ..., z_{p-H+1}$ will be elected by the maximum pooling method, which will finally provide a new vector z:

$$z = \max(z_j) \tag{5.16}$$

Bidirectional gated recurrent unit

A type of RNN is referred to as GRU. Similar to LSTM, GRU is considered a remedy for long-term memory retention and gradient issues in backpropagation. RNNs perform recursion in the evolutionary sequence direction with sequential input data, where each neurone is interconnected in a chain. Neurones can simultaneously receive information from other neurones and their own past states due to the presence of cyclic factors in the hidden layer. Consequently, RNN exhibits both parameter sharing and memory sharing. Furthermore, RNN excels at acquiring nonlinear characteristics from sequential data. LSTM is proposed as a remedy for the vanishing gradient issue in RNNs and its inadequacy in learning long-term historical dependencies. LSTM can learn correlations between short-term and long-term sequential data. Subsequently, GRU was developed to address the challenges of LSTM, including its slower convergence rate and unnecessary parameterisation. A variation of LSTM with reduced parameters is termed GRU, which demonstrates enhanced convergence speed while retaining the superior learning capacity of LSTM. The internal elements of GRU comprise the update gate and the reset gate.

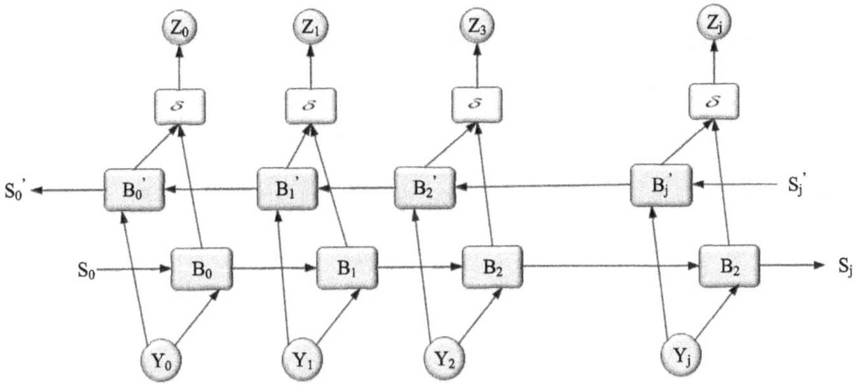

Figure 5.4. Structure of BiGRU

Figure 5.4 illustrates the configuration of the BiGRU. It emphasises its internal elements, including the update gate and reset gate. This architecture enables the BiGRU to efficiently regulate information flow by discerning which features to eliminate or preserve. Consequently, tackling the issues of long-term dependency in sequential data. Unlike LSTM, GRU replaces the forgetting gate and input gate of an LSTM with an update gate. The update gate determines the influence of the output data from hidden layer neurones at a previous time on the neurones in the current hidden layer. A greater updating gate value indicates a larger degree of effect. Unlike LSTM, GRU replaces the forgetting gate and input gate of LSTM with an update gate. The update gate determines the influence of the output data from hidden layer neurones at a previous time on the neurones in the current hidden layer. A greater updating gate value corresponds to a larger degree of influence. The extent of neurone output disregard in the preceding hidden layer is defined by the resetting gate. The subsequent formula can be utilised to delineate the hidden layer unit B:

$$Z_u = \delta(w_Z \cdot [H_{u-1}, y_u]) \tag{5.17}$$

$$R_u = \delta(w_R \cdot [H_{u-1}, y_u]) \tag{5.18}$$

$$\widetilde{H}_u = \tanh(w[R_u * H_{u-1}, y_u]) \tag{5.19}$$

$$H_u = (1 - Z_u) * H_{u-1} + Z_u * \widetilde{H}_u \tag{5.20}$$

where, δ indicates the Sigmoid function, $\tanh$ specifies the hyperbolic tangent function, and Z_u and R_u specify the updating and resetting gates. w_R, v_R, w_Z, v_Z, and v signify all the matrices of training parameter. The resetting gate R_u, the input Y_u at the current instant, the output H_{u-1} of the hidden layer neuron at the preceding moment, and the training parameter matrices v and u work together to establish the candidate activation state $\widetilde{H}_u$ at the present moment.

In order to learn the deep features for women nutrition recommendation, BiGRU network is better to learn the relationship among current, past and future influencing factors. It is computed as

$$z_2 = g(vB_2 + v'B_2') \tag{5.21}$$

and B_2' are computed using

$$B_2 = g(wB_1 + uy_2) \tag{5.22}$$

$$B_2' = g(w'B_3' + uy_2) \tag{5.23}$$

The hidden layer value S_u in the forward calculation is associated to S_{u-1}. The value of hidden layer S_u in the reverse computation is associated to S_{u-1}. The sum of the reverse and forward computations governs the final result. The calculation procedure of bidirectional RNN is given as follows:

$$O_u = g(vS_u + v'S_u') \tag{5.24}$$

$$S_u = f(uy_u + wS_{u-1}) \tag{5.25}$$

$$S_u' = f(u'y_u + w'S_{u-1}') \tag{5.26}$$

The cross-entropy (CE) loss function is employed for the classification problem in the neural network. The hyper-parameters of the classification model is tuned by the provided metaheuristic algorithm by minimizing the loss function.

Cross attention mechanism

Attention mechanism (AM) is aimed at minimising the impact of irrelevant information and maximising the information on the relevant information so as to make recommendations on health nutrients and make optimal decisions. The AM is useful in two areas, foremost, it is able to automatically detect the local data that need to be incorporated into the global input. Secondly, it assigns more processing capabilities to activities that are critical. These two advantages may influence the use of AM to improve local information attributes. The aim of the task and attention region are different. There is ideal utilisation of the critical information when the local data is gathered. The attention network is articulated in the following way:

$$Z_u = g(z_{u-1}, m_{u-1}, D_u) \tag{5.27}$$

where, Z_u characterizes the output of AM at instant u, g specifies the dense layer, Z_{u-1} implies the output of AM at time $u-1$, and m_{u-1} designates the label at moment $u-1$.

$$D_u = \sum_{k=1}^{U_y} b_{uk} i_k \tag{5.28}$$

where, D_u characterizes the output of succeeding phase, i_k implies the kth input of AM, and b_{uk} designates the attention weight,.

$$b_{uk} = \frac{\exp(e_{uk})}{\sum_{l=1}^{U_y} \exp(e_{ul})} \tag{5.29}$$

$$e_{uk} = h(z_{u-1}, i_k) = w \times \tanh(X \times i_k + v \times Z_{u-1} + c) \tag{5.30}$$

where, h is employed to compute the extent of association between Z_{u-1} and i_k, and b_{uk} designates the degree to which the current AM is allied and k^{th} input. More attention is engrossed on the component when the extent of association is greater.

Cross-attention: The conventional AM, which a one-way AM that allocated weight to attention in only one direction, lost a number of distinctive variables. The summing of weight matrix via elements and the weight maximization strategy are the two tandem weight allocation techniques used by the HABi-ConGRNet. It also utilizes the cross-attention mechanism (CrAM). The weight coefficients are first calculated in the vertical and horizontal directions using the CrAM. The structure of CrAM is provided in Figure 5.5. The CrAM allocates attention weights in both vertical and horizontal directions. By obtaining the most representative features, this dual-directional method progresses feature extraction. The mechanism improves the model's performance through the usage of weight addition and maximization methods. The schematic demonstrates how the weights are computed and applied to the input data. This mechanism reduces information loss and guarantees effective feature mining.

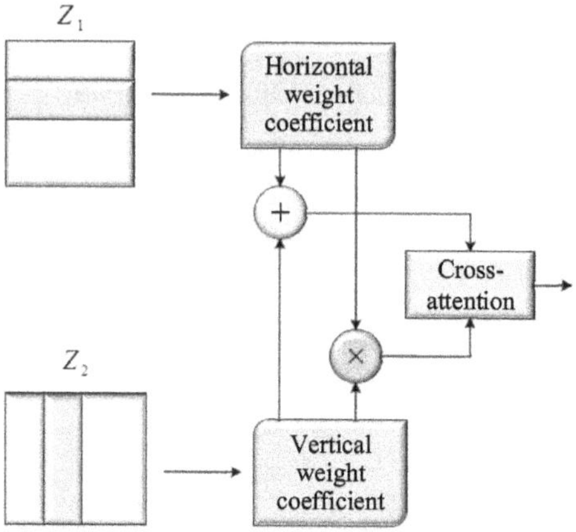

Figure 5.5 Structure of CrAM

The resulting element weights are then increased in two perpendicular directions for strengthening the features, and a maximizing technique is employed to get maximum weight coefficients. As a result, the combined result of two methods has been gained. Weights are multiplied and maximized using the expression below.

$$Z_{uk} = \sum_{k=1}^{U_y} \frac{\exp(e_{uk})}{\sum_{l=1}^{U_y} \exp(e_{ul})} i_k \tag{5.31}$$

$$Add = (Z_1 + Z_2) \tag{5.32}$$

$$Max = (Z_1, Z_2) \tag{5.33}$$

$$CrAM = concatenate[Z_1, Z_2, Add, Max] \tag{5.34}$$

where, Z_1 designates the weight coefficient of vertical AM, Z_2 describes the weight coefficient of horizontal AM, Add signifies the weight coefficients summation and Max specifies the maximization of weight coefficients. CrAM in HABi-ConGRNet assigns weight values to the output of the feature map's BiGRU from two dimensions that are not parallel to each other. Then, it combines those feature maps with the original feature map by maximising and adding the weight values. This shows the most important features and makes the best use of the resources provided by the computer.

5.3 HYPER-PARAMETER TUNING

Hyper-parameter tune-up is considered to be the procedure of the choice of the best values of the parameters in the classification model of the proposed OdriHDL method. To optimise the classification performance using the proposed OdriHDL approach, the Greylag Goose Optimisation Algorithm (GGOA) is used to optimise the hyper-parameters. GGOA is based on the dynamic characteristics of goose. It starts with the creation of people randomly, each of whom is a possible solution to a specific issue. These individuals are then broken down into exploration and exploitation groups, the amount in each group being dynamically adjusted according to the success of the ideal solution. This helps to avoid any trapping of the algorithm on local optima and makes the exploration of the solution space effective. In hyper-parameter tuning, the geese are the hyper-parameters, and the optimal parameter values are the best.

The GGOA exploration algorithm is aimed at finding intriguing regions within the search space and preventing stalling on local optima by moving towards the ideal solution. It is done using accurate equations to change the position of the agents through iterations. The basic form of the equation of GGOA of changing the position of the agents is as follows:

$$Y(u+1) = Y'(u) - B\left|D.Y'(u) - Y(u)\right| \tag{5.35}$$

where, $Y(u)$ designates the position of the agent at iteration u, and $Y'(u)$ designates the position of the best solution (leader). During iterations, the GGOA utilizes the following equations to update vectors B and D, which are designated as $B = 2b.s_1 - b$ and $D = 2.s_2$, respectively. The parameter b varies linearly from 2 to 0. s_1 and s_2 are randomly altering values within $[0,1]$.

The following equation, which considers three randomly chosen search agents (paddings), designated as $Y_{Paddle,1}$, $Y_{Paddle,2}$, and $Y_{Paddle,3}$, is incorporated into the algorithm to further enhance exploration:

$$Y(u+1) = W_1 Y_{Paddle,1} + ZW_2(Y_{Paddle,2} - Y_{Paddle,3}) + (1-Z)W_3(Y - Y_{Paddle,1}) \tag{5.36}$$

where, W_1, W_2, and W_3 are updated within $[0,2]$, and Z is minimized exponentially depending on $Z = 1-(u/u_{Max})^2$, where u_{Max} represents the maximum number of iterations.

In the second updating stage, when $s_3 \geq 0.5$, the values of b and vector B are decreased:

$$Y(u+1) = W_4 \left|Y'(u) - Y(u)\right| e^{cm} \cos(2\pi m) + 2W_1(s_4 + s_5)Y'(u) \quad (5.37)$$

where, W_4 updates within $[0,2]$, m specifies the random number in $[-1,1]$, s_4 and s_5 update within [0,1], and c indicates a constant.

The exploitative part of GGOA is all about making already existing solutions better based on how well they work (Mean Square Error (MSE)). There are two different ways to reach the goals of exploitation. These tactics work together to make the solution better overall.

Moving in the direction of best solution: In order to direct individuals $(Y_{nonsentry,1})$ toward the predicted prey position, the algorithm utilizes the following equation, which is guided by three sentry solutions ($Y_{sentry,1}, Y_{sentry,2}$ and $Y_{sentry,3}$).

$$Y_1 = Y_{sentry,1} - B_1 . \left|D_1 . Y_{sentry,1} - Y\right| \quad (5.38)$$

$$Y_2 = Y_{sentry,2} - B_2 . \left|D_1 . Y_{sentry,2} - Y\right| \quad (5.39)$$

$$Y_3 = Y_{sentry,3} - B_3 . \left|D_1 . Y_{sentry,3} - Y\right| \quad (5.40)$$

where, D_1, D_2 and D_3 are calculated as $D = 2s_2$, and B_1, B_2 and B_3 are computed as $B = 2b.s_1 - b$. The average of three solutions, Y_1, Y_2 and Y_3, is used to define the updated locations for the population, $Y(u+1)$ as follows:

$$Y(u+1) = \frac{1}{3}\sum_{j=1}^{3} Y_j \quad (5.41)$$

Searching the area around optimal solution: In this tactic, individuals look for improvements in areas close to the optimal solution. The equation for updating a position is offered by:

$$Y(u+1) = Y(u) + E(1+a) * W * (Y - Y_{fok}) \quad (5.42)$$

where, W represents an additional exploration parameter, E resembles a constant, a states a parameter computed by the number of iterations, and Y_{fok} indicates the optimal response (leader).

These methods let people move their positions closer to more promising sections of the search space, which lets the GGOA keep improving solutions. Algorithm 1 shows the pseudocode for GGOA that can help you find the best parameters.

Pseudocode of GGOA for hyper-parameter tuning

Start

Initialize the population of GGOA $Y_j(j=1,2,3,....,p)$, fitness function F_p, iteration u_{Max}

Initialize the parameters of GGOA

Compute the fitness function F_p for each agent Y_j

Set $Q=$position of best agent

Update solutions in exploration group (p_1) and exploitation group (p_2)

While $u \leq u_{Max}$ do

For $(j=1:j<p_1+1)$ do

If $(u\%2==0)$ then

If $(s_3<0.5)$ then

If $(|B|<1)$ then

Update search agent location as $Y(u+1)=Y'(u)-B|D.Y'(u)-Y(u)|$

Else

Choose three random search agents $Y_{Paddle,1}$, $Y_{Paddle,2}$, and $Y_{Paddle,3}$

Update Z through exponential form of $Z=1-(u/u_{Max})^2$

Update current search agent location as $Y(u+1)=W_1 Y_{Paddle,1}+ZW_2(Y_{Paddle,2}-Y_{Paddle,3})+(1-Z)W_3(Y-Y_{Paddle,1})$

End if

Else

Update current search agent location as $Y(u+1) = W_4 \left| Y'(u) - Y(u) \right| e^{cm} \cos(2\pi m) + 2W_1 (s_4 + s_5) Y'(u)$
End if
Else
Update individual location as $Y(u+1) = Y(u) + E(1+a) * W * (Y - Y_{fok})$
End if
End for
Compute fitness function
Update the parameters
Set $u = u+1$
End if
End while
Return best agent Q

Table 5.1. Hyper parameter settings of OdriHDL model

Parameters	**Values**
Max epochs	100
Learning rate	0.01
Mini batch size	32
Optimizer	GGOA
Loss function	CE
Drop out	0.5
Training data	80%
Testing data	20%

The OdriHDL model gives you personalised nutrition advice in real time to help you reduce your symptoms and enhance your health during your period in table 5.1. The next sections also give information on how to gather data, evaluate performance, and set up metrics for the OdriHDL model for women's nutrition advice during their menstrual cycle.

Data collection

Real-time data for testing was gathered through comprehensive consultations with advisors specialising in menstrual health and nutrition. The correlation of specific nutrient recommendations to symptoms, such as severe cramping, was facilitated by professional guidance. The dataset consists of 2000 samples utilised for training deep learning models. Menstrual symptoms such as mood fluctuations, cephalalgia, abdominal distension, lethargy, acne, mammary tenderness, and cramps, along with individual factors including stress levels, age, and Body Mass Index (BMI), are regarded as inputs. The anticipated nutrient guidelines for iron, magnesium, calcium, and vitamin D are classified as moderate, low, or high. Each dataset includes a unique identifier, BMI (ranging from 18.5 to 30.5), age of individuals between 18 and 50, stress level from 0 (no stress) to 3 (severe stress), menstrual cycle day (1 to 28), and cycle phase classified as follicular, menstruation, luteal, or ovulation. Furthermore, symptoms associated with the menstrual cycle, including mood swings, headaches, bloating, exhaustion, acne, breast tenderness, and cramps, are assessed on a scale from 0 to 3, where 0 signifies absence of symptoms, 1 shows mild symptoms, 2 denotes moderate symptoms, and 3 reflects severe symptoms. The anticipated nutrition encompasses the consumption of calcium (mg/day), iron (mg/day), magnesium (mg/day), and vitamin D (IU/day). Furthermore, these nutritional requirements are categorised as moderate, low, or high.

For iron, the low classification denotes a demand of 0–10 mg daily, the moderate classification corresponds to 10–18 mg, and the high classification signifies a need beyond 18 mg. For calcium, a low classification signifies a consumption of 0-500 mg daily, moderate implies 500-1000 mg, and high refers to an intake over 1000 mg. For magnesium, low intake is defined as 0-200 mg, moderate intake as 200-400 mg, and high intake as over 400 mg. Finally, for vitamin D, low denotes an intake of 0-1000 IU per day, moderate indicates an intake of 1000-2000 IU, and high characterises an intake above 2000 IU. The OdriHDL model is trained using the provided data to prescribe women's nutritional requirements for magnesium, calcium, iron, and vitamin D, taking into account their menstrual phase, symptoms, and personal health information.

5.4 HYPOTHESIS AND LIMITATION

Clinical trials and observational research have traditionally been fundamental to the nutrition business; however, the advent of AI has supplanted them. These technologies, encompassing data analysis, deep learning, and machine learning, has the ability to identify patterns, generate valuable insights, and uncover complex relationships within data. This section discusses the OdriHDL model, which is aimed to provide personalised diet recommendations. The OdriHDL model utilises HABi-ConGRNet to evaluate intricate patterns in nutritional requirements by taking into account personal health measurements and menstruation symptoms. The model incorporates extensive data pre-processing, feature extraction utilising LSAENet, and a resilient classification methodology to enhance recommendation precision. The quantitative results indicate a 97.52% accuracy rate, showcasing its proficiency in classifying and recommending vital nutrients, surpassing the performance of current RNN, CNN-LSTM, CNN-BiLSTM, and attention GRU models, which have achieved accuracy rates between 85% and 92%. The recall of 96.91% and precision of 97.82% underscore the model's dependability in precisely assessing the dietary requirements of women. Furthermore, to ascertain the model's superiority, the proposed OdriHDL is compared with leading approaches in Table 5.2 The present LSTM utilised for patient diet guidance has demonstrated superior performance; however, it has experienced overfitting and insufficient convergence. The K-clique integrated GRU classifier has achieved lower accuracy. The suggested OdriHDL model has achieved superior accuracy and effectively addresses overfitting concerns.

Table 5.2 Comparison of proposed with state-of-the-art methods

Method	Dataset used	Accuracy (%)	Field
LSTM	Health-based medical dataset	97.74	Patient diet recommendation
K-clique integrated GRU classifier	Data collected from internet and hospitals	Close to 96	Patient diet recommendation
Proposed	Data collected from open source and Kaggle and PubMed	97.52	Women nutrition recommendation

This demonstrates the potential of the OdriHDL model for practical application in health technology. The principal benefit of the OdriHDL model is its integration of an advanced feature extraction framework using LSAENet, enhancing the model's ability to discern intricate correlations between nutritional needs and menstruation symptoms. Moreover, the application of HABi-ConGRNet facilitates a deeper comprehension of data, leading to improved classification performance. The model's optimisation also leads to decreased training duration and expedited convergence, enhancing its efficiency for practical applications. Notwithstanding the enhancements, the suggested approach presents specific constraints. The dependence on particular data can restrict the model's generalisability, since it may fail to encompass varied experiences and nutritional requirements. Furthermore, the intricacy of design presents challenges regarding interpretability and ease of implementation in practical environments, while yet demonstrating potential for accuracy.

5.5 SUMMARY

This chapter delineated the conceptual foundation and methodological framework for the proposed Optimization-driven Hybrid Deep Learning (OdriHDL) model, designed to deliver precise and personalised nutrition recommendations for women during various phases of the menstrual cycle. The research challenge was established by highlighting the inadequacies of current systems in accommodating dynamic physiological changes and articulating the goal to remedy this deficiency using an adaptive, data-driven methodology. The chapter thereafter described the research objectives and articulated the scope and limitations of the investigation. The proposed methodology encompasses several stages: data pre-processing to guarantee high-quality and structured input; feature extraction employing a Layered Sparse Autoencoder Network (LSAENet) to identify intricate relationships between menstrual symptoms and nutrient needs; classification through a Hybrid Attention-based Bidirectional Convolutional Greylag Goose Gated Recurrent Network (HABi-ConGRNet) to model spatial-temporal dependencies; and hyperparameter optimisation utilising the Greylag Goose Optimisation Algorithm (GGOA) to improve model accuracy and minimise error rates. The OdriHDL model integrates advanced feature learning, hybrid deep learning architecture, and metaheuristic optimisation to provide stage-specific, accurate, and dependable nutrient recommendations for calcium, iron, magnesium, and vitamin D, thereby enhancing menstrual health management relative to current methodologies.

www.ingramcontent.com/pod-product-compliance
Lightning Source LLC
LaVergne TN
LVHW010738061126
851857LV00014B/1547
* 9 7 8 1 9 6 2 1 1 6 4 8 0 *